hn A. Graziano Memorial Library
Samuel Merritt University
400 Hawthorne Avenue
Oakland CA 94609
510-869-8900

WB
18.2
S83
2005

SURVIVAL GUIDE TO THE

USMLE

STEP 2CS

D0743423

MAY 1 8 2009

SURVIVAL GUIDE TO THE
USMLE
STEP 2CS

Vivek Subbiah, MD

Resident, Internal Medicine and Pediatrics
Case Western Reserve University School of Medicine
MetroHealth Medical Center
Cleveland, Ohio

Rishi Sharma, MD

Research Associate
Hematology/Oncology
Northwestern University The Feinberg School of Medicine
Chicago, Illinois

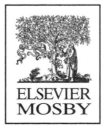

ELSEVIER
MOSBY

**ELSEVIER
MOSBY**

An Affiliate of Elsevier

The Curtis Center
170 S Independence Mall W 300E
Philadelphia, Pennsylvania 19106

SURVIVAL GUIDE TO THE USMLE STEP 2CS   ISBN 0-323-03585-X

Copyright © 2005 by Mosby, Inc.

All rights reserved. No part of this publication may be reproduced or transmitted in any form or by any means, electronic or mechanical, including photocopy, recording, or any information storage and retrieval system, without permission in writing from the publisher.

NOTICE

Medicine is an ever-changing field. Standard safety precautions must be followed, but as new research and clinical experience broaden our knowledge, changes in treatment and drug therapy may become necessary or appropriate. Readers are advised to check the most current product information provided by the manufacturer of each drug to be administered to verify the recommended dose, the method and duration of administration, and contraindications. It is the responsibility of the licensed prescriber, relying on experience and knowledge of the patient, to determine dosages and the best treatment for each individual patient. Neither the publisher nor the authors assume any liability for any injury and/or damage to persons or property arising from this publication.

Acquisitions Editor: Linda Belfus
Developmental Editor: Stan Ward

Printed in the United States of America

Last digit is the print number: 9 8 7 6 5 4 3 2 1

DEDICATION

To my mother Mullai, my father Subbiah,

my sister Niveditha, my grandfather Prof. S. N. Chokkalingam,

who has inspired me by authoring more than 100 books,

and my grandmother Thayammal.

Vivek Subbiah

To my mother Rachna, my father Bhagwan,

and my brother Neil.

Rishi Sharma

PREFACE

Congratulations on being one step closer to becoming a doctor in the United States. We are delighted to bring you the first edition of *The Survival Guide to the USMLE Step 2CS*. Given the ever-evolving medical field, we wanted to provide the quintessentials needed for more than passing the USMLE Step 2-CS. Remember—it's a jungle out there! This *Survival Guide* is the most effective and efficient way to prepare for the exam.

First-hand information is provided in a friendly, simple format. This honest student-to-student guide saves you a great deal of time. And remember: saving time + effort + money = success. The insider tips and tricks will give you an edge over the competition. In the end, the jungle turns out to be an amusement park.

The *Survival Guide* is a step-by-step approach to instant success. The time-tested mnemonics, the tips for the physical exam and patient counseling and closure, and the guide to the write-up of patient notes are provided in an easy-to-read and unique layout. Included are 100 common exam presentations, along with differential diagnoses, investigations, red flags, focused history, and targeted physical examinations.

This book would not have been possible without the efforts of Linda Belfus, Vice-President of Elsiever. We apreciate this opportunity to share our knowledge with the future generations of medical students.

We also gratefully acknowledge the invaluable contributions of Raj Joshi, future MD, St. Louis University, who provided the illustrations.

In addition we would like to thank Doctors Swaminatha Mahadevan (Stanford University Medical Center, Palo Alto, CA); Holly B. Perzy, David J. Mansour, Ben Brouhard, Alfred F. Connors, Jr., Michael J. McFarlane, Robert C. Cohn, Abdullah Gori, Robert Needlman, Rupesh Raina, and David C. Kaelber (Case Western Reserve University, MetroHealth, Cleveland, OH); Ashok Agarwal (Cleveland Clinic Foundation, Cleveland OH); Thanikachalam, K.V. Somasundaram, V. Gurumurthy, and TR. Gopalan (Sri Ramachandra Medical College and R.I., Harvard Medical International Associated Institution, India); C.S. Meenakshi (King Institute); Charles Bennet (Northwestern University, Chicago) Rashmi Kapur and Nicholas Vogel (University of Illinois at Chicago); Rene Archilla and Abbassam Habbal (University of Illinois at Chicago, Christ Medical Center); Krishna Chaitanya (University of Missouri, Kansas City); Jayant Malhotra and Veerpal Singh (Northwestern University, Evanston)

Special thanks to Barbara Wada, Elizabeth While, Thiru and Radha Venkatachalam.

Finally, we hope that this edition will provide our readers with enough useful and up-to-date information to pass the USMLE Step 2-CS with flying colors. Comments and recommendations for future editions are always welcome. Please e-mail us at USMLE2CS@yahoo.com and give us your input.

VIVEK SUBBIAH, MD

RISHI SHARMA, MD

CONTENTS

PREFACE
vii

INTRODUCTION
xi

1 INTRODUCTION AND FREQUENTLY ASKED QUESTIONS
1

2 VIRTUAL EXAM
5

3 HISTORY TAKING
9

4 THE PHYSICAL EXAM
19

5 COUNSELING, TACKLING DIFFICULT SITUATIONS, COMMUNICATING BAD NEWS
31

6 CLOSING THE ENCOUNTER
35

7 THE PATIENT NOTE
37

8 65 SAMPLE CASES
41

9 35 PRACTICE CASES
103

10 ANSWERS FOR THE 35 PRACTICE CASES
121

11 Model Case
143

12 Appendix
151

Index
159

INTRODUCTION

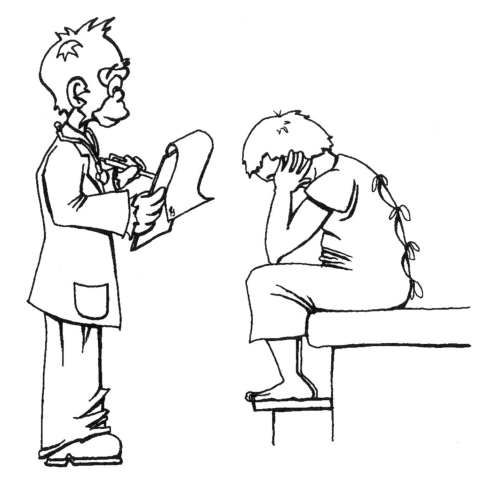

As for the Olympics or any sporting event, we have included a mascot for you. Dr. Vix will be your guide through this book. Think of the exam as a game, and Dr. Vix will lead you to a gold medal in this clinical "Skillympics."

INTRODUCTION AND FREQUENTLY ASKED QUESTIONS

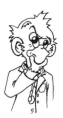

The United States Medical Licensing Exam Step 2 Clinical Skills (USMLE Step 2-CS) effectively tests communication skills in a one-on-one relationship between the doctor and the patient in a hospital environment. Although the exam does not use actual patients, the student is tested through a series of standardized patients who simulate specific complaints. Until January 2004, only foreign medical graduates were required to take this exam for certification in the United States. Because of the increasing demands of the doctor-patient relationship, however, starting with the graduating class of 2005 this exam will be mandatory for all U.S. medical school graduates.

Although the number one factor in physician job dissatisfaction is the poor quality of the doctor-patient relationship, few institutions emphasize this aspect of medical practice. Surprisingly, most physicians have never been observed during a patient interview by someone who is an expert in the process and who can give the right feedback.

Various organizations are concerned with research on and education about the physician-patient interview. In the United States, these institutions include the American Academy on Physician and Patient, and in the United Kingdom, the Medical Interview Teachers Association.

In addition, the Association of Standardized Patient Educators provides support, resources, and educational opportunities to medical educators involved in standardized patient methodology, from deans and medical directors to teaching and support faculty, program coordinators, and standardized patient trainers.

FREQUENTLY ASKED QUESTIONS

What is the Step 2-CS?

The Step 2-CS focuses on physician-patient communication skills. Formerly known as the CSA (Clinical Skills Assessment), it was a requirement for foreign medical graduates to obtain full medical licensure in the United States. Starting with the graduating year of 2005, all medical students who plan to pursue graduate medical education will be required to take the Step 2-CS.

The exam focuses on different aspects of the doctor-patient interview. The diagnosis is the least important aspect of the exam. Instead, the student is expected to formulate a differential diagnosis. The student will be assessed on his or her overall approach to a given set of symptoms, with the assessment including every aspect of the interview:

doctor introduction, detailed history taking, performance of a properly focused physical examination, counseling, provision of advice on treatment, and closure. In addition, the student will be required to write or type the patient note, which may include a maximum of five possible diagnoses and five different investigations.

Do we get real patients?

The answer is yes and no. You will see a standardized patient (SP). As H.S. Barrows observed in *Simulated (Standardized) Patients and Other Human Simulations* (1987): "The SP is a person who has been carefully coached to simulate an actual patient so accurately that the simulation cannot be detected by a skilled clinician. In performing the simulation, the SP presents the gestalt of the patient being simulated; not just the history, but the body language, the physical findings, and the emotional and personality characteristics as well."

Do SPs have any positive symptoms?

An ordinary patient may not be able to simulate splenomegaly, but a patient with splenomegaly can quite possibly be trained as an SP. Certain signs (e.g., a heart murmur) cannot be mimicked unless the SP already has them. But signs such as hyperreflexia or paralysis can be mimicked.

Where do I get more information about the exam?
What are the prerequisites for the exam?
How do I register for, schedule, or reschedule the exam?
What are the accommodations for examinees with documented disabilities?

Information pertaining to the Step 2-CS is available on the following websites:

www.usmle.org
www.ecfmg.org
www.nbme.org
www.fsmb.org

Where is this exam offered?

Philadelphia, Pennsylvania
Atlanta, Georgia
Los Angeles, California
Chicago, Illinois
Houston, Texas

How is the Step 2-CS scored?

Performance on the Step 2-CS will be reported as pass or fail. Examinees who fail will receive performance profiles showing the relative strengths and weaknesses of the examinee's performance across the components of the Step 2-CS.
Three primary components of a Step 2-CS exam are assessed:

1. Data-gathering skills, including history-taking and physical examination skills, and completion of a patient note
2. Communication/interpersonal skills
3. Proficiency in spoken English

A passing performance on all three components in a single administration is required to obtain the overall designation of passing the Step 2-CS.

Is there a dress code for the exam?

Technically, there is no dress code for the exam. However, we strongly suggest the business/professional dress code. You may look great in an unbuttoned plaid shirt and rolled-up jeans or in clothes that you could wear to go dancing in right after the exam, but you probably should rethink such outfits. You either are a doctor or will be a doctor; therefore, you should dress professionally.

THE THOUGHT PROCESS REQUIRED FOR THE EXAM

- For any given symptom, the thought process should begin with a set of possible diagnoses (the differential diagnoses) and possible investigations.
- After taking a detailed history, you should perform a focused physical exam *only* on the relevant systems. Advise and counsel the patient about the differential diagnoses and the possible investigations that you plan to do, just as if this were a real patient encounter.
- Write or type the patient note.

The importance of knowing the differential diagnoses and appropriate investigations for all possible cases that may be presented to you cannot be overemphasized. The Step 2-CS is a race against time, and the best method of preparation is to know these two aspects very well. The differential diagnoses and investigations should account for 50% of your write-up; having this knowledge at your fingertips will also help you in the physical examination and counseling of the patient.

Sample Case

A 57-year-old man arrives in the ED with chest pain for the past 3 hours.

- First think of a possible list of five relevant diagnoses:

    1. Myocardial infarction
    2. Pericarditis
    3. Gastroesophageal reflux disease (GERD)
    4. Unstable angina
    5. Pneumonia

- At the back of your mind you should also be thinking of possible investigations that would exclude one or another diagnosis, such as electrocardiography (ECG), chest x-ray, or assessment of cardiac enzymes.
- Take a complete history of the patient's presenting illness, past medical history, and social history.
- Perform a targeted cardiovascular examination and a respiratory examination.
- Advise and counsel the patient about the differential diagnoses, what the patient needs to do, what you are going to do for the patient, and the prognosis of the disease.
- Leave the room and write down all of your findings.

Now you have finished.

VIRTUAL EXAM 2

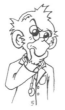

Congratulations! Taking this exam is a huge achievement in itself. You must try to stay calm and confident about the entire exam. Efficient preparation is the key to success. The entire exam is well organized and efficiently timed. The Step 2-CS proctors are friendly and very helpful in guiding you through the exam. So just kick back and relax while we guide you through the Step 2-CS.

THE DAY OF THE EXAM

You must arrive no later than one-half hour before your scheduled exam time. The first step is registration. You have to present your appointment schedule permit and one form of government-issued identification, such as a passport or U.S. driver's license. You will be issued an identification badge and a number to pin on your left upper arm. Then you must sign a confidentiality agreement. Basically, the agreement ensures that you do not leak the contents of the exam to future test-takers. It is breach of agreement if you reveal any information about the exam to anyone via the Internet, oral discussions, or publications. The proctors then give you a sheet of scratch paper for each case that you will see. This allows you to scribble notes during the encounter. Double-check that you have a sheet of scratch paper designated for each patient encounter. A pen also will be issued. Make sure that you do not write anything on the scratch paper before the actual exam begins.

Once everyone is registered, you will be taken to an orientation room, where you will leave all of your belongings except your lab coat, stethoscope, identification, and yourself! Everything else is stored in a cubicle to which you will have access only at the end of the exam. Make sure that you leave all of your notes (including this book!), your cell phone (switched off), and any other electronic gadgets in the locker. Any break in conduct will lead to review. At any of the USMLE exams, someone is always watching. Do not think that you can get past the video monitors located just about every step of the way. You are a professional, and you are expected to act accordingly.

ORIENTATION

A video presentation follows. Any new information about the exam will be given to you at this time. The proctors will then introduce to you the instruments available in each examination room. They will allot you an ample amount of time to become familiar with the instruments, understand how to elevate and bring down the examination table, and relax. Available instruments include an ophthalmoscope, Snellen chart, two tuning forks with different frequencies, cotton swabs, cotton balls, tooth picks, tongue depressors, reflex hammer, otoscope, sphygmomanometer, drape, latex gloves, and ample soap and paper towels by the wash basin. Any doubts or questions you have can be cleared up at this time. Don't bombard the proctors with insignificant questions—make sure that your questions are really sensible.

You should know your tools. Some people confuse an otoscope with an ophthalmoscope.

THE ACTUAL EXAM

You will see a long, narrow corridor with more than 12 doors on each side. It looks much like the inside of a subway train! Between the doors, against the wall, are small workstations at which you will be required to write or type your patient notes. Each door has a plastic box with a laterally sliding cover that contains the patient information. The information includes the patient's name and age, the setting (ED, office), the patient's chief complaints and vital signs, and the task to be performed.

At the start of the exam you will hear a faint announcement, "SP, please prepare." Don't do anything yet. Approximately 2 minutes later you will hear a louder announcement: "Doctors, you may begin." At this point your master clock begins. You have 15 minutes for the patient encounter and 10 minutes to write the patient note. If you complete the patient encounter in less than 15 minutes, you may leave the examination room to start writing the patient note. Once you leave the examination room, you are not allowed to return for any reason. If you left any papers or instruments in the room, inform the proctor, who will retrieve them for you. But if you exceed the 15 minutes, a proctor will knock, enter, and escort you outside the examination room. Don't wait for the proctor to pull you out!

After the announcement, "Doctors, you may begin," open the sliding window on the door box and read the patient information. The time you spend reading the patient information counts in your 15 minutes, but do not rush. Once you enter the examination room, the SP will occupy your time. Therefore, while you are still outside the examination room, allow yourself about 45 seconds to gather your thoughts, think of possible diagnoses and investigations, and consider what systems to examine. Some students might enter the room immediately—don't worry about them. Also, at this time you may start to write on the scratch paper that the proctors provided. Jot down the name of the patient and any relevant history items. If you miss any information in the door box, do not panic; there is a second copy of the information in the room.

The SP may be standing, or sitting on the examination table, or lying down wearing a gown. In the room, apart from the examination table, sink, and instruments, there is a stool on which a drape is usually placed. Use the drape to cover the patient if needed. There will also be a computer for the SP to grade your performance once you leave the room.

During your 15 minutes with the patient, another alarm will sound at the 10-minute point, indicating that only 5 minutes are left. At this point you should ideally be completing the physical examination of the SP or just starting the counseling portion of the exam.

After your closing statements (or after your 15 minutes have elapsed), you will leave (or be escorted from) the examination room and return to the corridor to start writing the patient note. Every room has a designated workstation. At this time you have two options: you can either hand-write the notes or type them on the computer. However, all of the patient note for a given encounter must be completed using one or the other option. Once you have chosen a particular method, you have to continue with it for that encounter. You have the option to change your method of write-up in the next patient encounter if necessary. You are allotted 10 minutes for the patient notes. After 8 minutes have elapsed, you will hear yet another alarm, indicating that only 2 minutes are left. If you left the examination room before the end of the 15-minute period, the time remaining can be added to your time for writing up that particular case. Remember that you do not have the option of returning to the examination room once you have left it. You are allowed, however, to look at the patient information listed on the door as needed, but make sure that you close the sliding door after you have finished. After 10 minutes have elapsed, continue to stay seated. The proctors will retrieve your notes as well as your scratch paper for that encounter.

The next encounter will start only after everyone has been positioned correctly. Reading the information in the door box, entering the room, examining and talking to the patient, and writing the note eventually becomes a mechanical routine, and the exam is over sooner than you may think. It is the first case that gives some students the jitters. But if you understand the information in this book, you will have nothing to worry about.

After the fourth or fifth patient encounter, there is a 30-minute break for a well-balanced lunch, the cost of which is included in the examination fee. Both vegetarian and nonvegetarian foods are served. Therefore, there is no need to bring any food products. We do recommend bringing an after-lunch breath mint for the SP's sake. After another three or four encounters there is another 15-minute break.

After your last case, you will be asked to fill out a brief questionnaire. Then you are done. Make sure that you gather all of your belongings before you leave. Now it's party time—you deserve it!

After a few days, don't forget to write us about anything that should be added to this book for your future colleagues. Also, feel free to send us your comments about this book at any time.

HISTORY TAKING

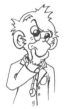

An important aspect of the Step 2-CS is the ability to elicit a proper, detailed history. Because of the time constraints, it is suggested that you memorize and practice the mnemonics provided in this chapter. Stress on the day of the exam may make you forget to do a lot of things you would have done had you not been in a testing environment. Use of mnemonics has been shown to increase the examinee's efficiency on the day of the exam.

Performing well on the history-taking component is determined by your use of spoken English, covering all the details necessary to construct a differential diagnosis, and making the SP as comfortable as possible.

Mnemonics makes life a lot easier on the day of the exam and hopefully will reduce some of your stress as you prepare for the exam.

HISTORY OF THE PRESENTING ILLNESS (HPI)

The HPI is the story behind the SP's chief complaint. It should be precise and at the same time complete. For any patient presenting with any type of pain, the following mnemonic is useful:

LIQOR DRAW (Drinking and drawing—what a combination!)

- **L** Location of the pain
- **I** Intensity
- **Q** Quality
- **O** Onset
- **R** Radiation

- **D** Duration
- **R** Relieving factors
- **A** Associated symptoms
- **W** Worsening factors

PAST MEDICAL HISTORY (PMH)

PACK BUSH SOS (MODELS) FTV
(PACK the BUSH beer SOS so we can watch the MODELS on FTV).

- **P** Previous history of the chief complaint
- **A** Allergies to any drugs, food, or any other specific allergen
- **C** Current medications
- **K** Known medical or surgical illness
- **B** Bowel changes + weight changes
- **U** Urinary complaints

- **S**   Sleep complaints
- **H**   History of previous hospitalizations

- **S**   Sexual history
- **O**   Obstetric and gynecologic history
- **S**   Social history

  - ➤ **M**   Marital
  - ➤ **O**   Occupation
  - ➤ **D**   Drugs, illicit
  - ➤ **E**   ETOH (alcohol)
  - ➤ **L**   Lifestyle
  - ➤ **S**   Smoking or chewing tobacco

- **F**   Family history relevant to patient's history
- **T**   Travel history
- **V**   Vaccinations

PEDIATRIC HISTORY

HPI plus ABCDEFGHIJK

- **A**   Antenatal history
- **B**   Birth history
- **C**   Cooking (feeding history)
- **D**   Developmental history
- **E**   Exposure history
- **F**   Family history
- **G**   Growth history/charts
- **H**   Hospitalization history
- **I**   Immunization history
- **J**   Just ask the name of the baby
- **K**   Kindly ask about the primary physician

TRAUMA HISTORY

If a trauma patient presents, make sure that you cover the following.

DR. ABCDEFGHI, then PMH

- **D**   Danger signs
- **R**   Responsiveness
- **A**   Airway
- **B**   Breathing
- **C**   Circulation
- **D**   Dermis (skin): bruises, cold, clammy
- **E**   Eye (e.g., dilated, constricted)
- **F**   Four extremities
- **G**   Gastrointestinal bleeding
- **H**   Hips
- **I**   Injuries (gross)

A case of domestic violence or abuse has to be SAVED:

- **S** Safety
- **A** Anxiety, stress
- **V** Violence, specific act of violence
- **E** Emergency plan
- **D** Domestic support system

PSYCHIATRIC HISTORY

CASE THIS IF MORPHINE JOKE, then PMH

- **C** Concentration
- **A** Appearance
- **S** Suicidal/homicidal ideation
- **E** Energy level

- **T** Time, place, and person orientation
- **H** Hallucinations
- **I** Interest in normal activities
- **S** Speech

- **I** Insight
- **F** Functionality/feelings

- **M** Memory
- **O** Optimism/pessimism
- **R** Reasoning
- **P** Paranoia
- **H** Hobbies
- **I** Irritability
- **N** Normal routine activities
- **E** Euphoria

- **J** Judgment
- **O** Outlook
- **K** Knowledge
- **E** Euthymia

DEPRESSION HISTORY

SIGE CAPS

- **S** Sleep
- **I** Interest
- **G** Guilt
- **E** Energy level

- **C** Concentration/memory
- **A** Appetite
- **P** Psychomotor retardation
- **S** Suicidal ideation

ACTIVITIES OF DAILY LIVING

SHEATH DRAFT

- **S**   Shopping
- **H**   Housekeeping
- **E**   Eating
- **A**   Ambulating
- **T**   Toileting
- **H**   Hygiene

- **D**   Dressing
- **R**   Remembering telephone numbers
- **A**   Accounting
- **F**   Food preparation
- **T**   Transportation

THE INTERVIEW

"The first impression is the best impression."

Generally speaking, one of the easiest cases presented to you on the Step 2-CS is a case of pain. On the doorway information, something like the following will be given:

Mr. Jim Adams presents to the ED. He is a 52-year-old man with pain in his chest for the past 4 hours.
   Vital signs:
- Blood pressure: 140/90 mm Hg
- Heart rate: 96 beats/minute
- Respiratory rate: 16 breaths/minute
- Temperature: 98.6°F

You are required to take a focused history, perform a physical exam, and evaluate Mr. Adams.

Introduction

This is an important part of the interview. Your introduction should be short and sweet. You must acknowledge the presence of the SP and his or her importance. According to the setting of the case (ED, hospital, office, or satellite health center), knock twice on the door and enter without waiting for a response. Greet the SP with a professional handshake. The proper handshake involves eye contact and a 3-second firm grip. Now let's see who can act better, the SP or you!

   "Good morning Mr. Adams (last name preferable). I am Dr. XYZ (your last name). I am the attending in the ED. It is nice to meet you. I'd like to ask you a few questions and then perform a physical exam. If you're feeling cold, would you like me to drape you? (This line shows compassion to the SP, indicating that you are interested in the SP's comfort.) *So, let's get started!"* (Show enthusiasm!)

Then ask an open-ended question:

"What brings you here today?"
or
"What caused you to come in today?"

As soon as the SP starts talking, make sure that you give him or her your <u>undivided attention.</u> Maintaining your posture and using proper eye contact increase the SP's compliance. Let the SP speak at his or her own pace. Show the SP that you are interested in everything the SP has to say.

Continue by asking:

> *"Is there anything else that you would like to add?"*
> or
> *"Can you tell me a little more about your chest pain?"*

Meanwhile, you should facilitate the interview with expressions such as "mm-hmmm," "go on," or "OK." You should also be <u>deciding what systems you need to evaluate and</u> <u>constructing a list of possible diagnoses and investigations.</u> Don't be afraid to write things down.

History of Presenting Illness

Use the mnemonic for the HPI, LIQOR DRAW (see p. 9):

- **L** *"Where is the pain/problem located?"*
  or
  "Can you show me with a finger where it hurts?"
- **I** *"On a scale from 1 through 10, 10 being the worst pain you've ever had and 1 being the least, can you grade your pain?"*
- **Q** *"Can you describe the pain?"*
  or
  "What does the pain feel like?"
  If the SP cannot find words to describe the pain, prompt him or her by using words such as stabbing, burning, crushing, sharp, dull, and so on.
- **O** *"When did this pain start?"*
- **R** *"Does it remain in the same place, or does it go anywhere else on your body?"* If yes, *"Where?"*

- **D** *"How long have you had this pain?"*
- **R** *"Have you noticed anything that makes the pain better?"*
- **A** *"Do you feel anything else that is associated with the pain?"*
  "Do you feel nauseated? Did you throw up? Do you have headache, fever, or shortness of breath?"
- **W** *"Have you noticed anything that makes the pain worse?"*

Past Medical History

Use the mnemonic for the PMH, PACK BUSH SOS (MODELS) FTV (see p. 9):

- **P** *"Have you ever experienced this type of pain in the past?"*
- **A** *"Are you allergic to any food or medication?"*
- **C** *"Are you currently on any medication?"*
- **K** *"Have you ever been diagnosed with any medical or surgical illnesses?"*
  "Do you have any other diseases such as high blood pressure (avoid using medical terms such as hypertension), *diabetes, or asthma?"*

- **B** *"Have you noticed any changes in your bowel habits?
  Any recent weight loss?"*
- **U** *"Have you had any problems urinating?"*
- **S** *"How are you sleeping?"*
- **H** *"Have you ever been hospitalized?"*

- **S** Before asking about the sexual history, state:
  "I'm now going to ask you some personal questions. Let me assure you that whatever we discuss will remain confidential. Is that alright with you?" Continue by asking,
  "Are you currently sexually active?"
  If yes:
    "Is it with one partner or multiple partners?"
    "Do you have sex with men, women, or both?"
    "Do you use any barrier method of contraception?"
    "Have you ever contracted a sexually transmitted disease?"
    "Have you ever been tested for HIV?"

  Note: Questions pertaining to STDs should be reserved for those with multiple sexual partners and those who fall into a high-risk group.

- **O** For female SPs only:
  "When was your last period?"
  "When was your first period?"
  "Are your periods regular?"
  "How many days are in your cycle?"
  "On a heavy day, how many pads do you use?"
  "Do you have cramps with your periods?" If yes, *"How bad are they?"*
  "Have you ever been pregnant?" If yes, *"How many times?"* *"How many children do you have?"* *"What was the mode of the delivery?"* *"Have you ever had a miscarriage?"*

- **S** *"I'm now going to ask you some questions about your personal life."*

  ➤ **(M)** *"Have you ever been married?"*
  ➤ **(O)** *"Are you currently employed?"*

  or
  "Tell me about what you do for a living."

  ➤ **(D)** *"Do you use any recreational or illicit drugs? Have you ever used intravenous drugs?"* If yes, *"What type of drugs and how often?"*

  Note: Try not to be judgmental. The term *abuse* should be avoided, and the term *use* should be used.

  ➤ **(E)** *"Do you drink alcohol?"* If yes, ask the quantity. If you suspect that the SP is an alcoholic, immediately ask the CAGE questions.

- **C** *"Have you ever felt the need to CUT down on your alcohol intake?"*
- **A** *"Do you feel ANNOYED when people tell you that you drink too much?"*
- **G** *"Do you feel GUILTY when you drink?"*
- **E** *"Have you ever taken a morning EYE-OPENER?"*

Note: Two yes answers are considered a positive screen. One yes answer should arouse suspicion of alcohol abuse.

➤ **(L)** *"Is there anything else about your lifestyle that I need to know?"*

➤ **(S)** *"Have you ever used tobacco? Either smoked or chewed?"* If yes, *"How many packs and for how many years have you been smoking?"*

Note: If the SP tells you that he or she quit some time ago, offer your congratulations and encourage the SP to keep up the good work.

● **F** *"Now I'd like to know a little about your family."*
"Has anyone in your family ever had the same symptoms that you are having now?"
"Has anyone in your family ever been diagnosed or treated for any medical or surgical illness?"

● **T** *"Have you traveled anywhere recently?"* If yes, *"Where?"*

Note: If the SP has traveled to an area of the world where certain diseases are more prevalent, ask if the SP took the proper precautions beforehand.

● **V** *"Is your vaccination schedule up to date?"*

Note: It is possible that the SP may respond by asking what types of vaccinations should be included. In this situation, it is essential that you know the proper vaccination schedules, along with the indications for and contraindications to the vaccines.

Pediatric History

The pediatric history may seem a challenge to some students, whereas in actuality it is another easy case. The reason is that there is probably no child present. Either one or both parents present the chief complaints of their child. Because no child is present, the entire 15 minutes may be spent taking the history of the child from the guardian. Do not forget that the number one investigation should include examination of the child.

Assuming that the mother of the child is presenting to you, use the mnemonic ABCDEFGHI (see p. 10):

● **A** *"Did you attend your prenatal visits on a regular basis?"*
"Was a sonogram performed at each visit?"
"Did you face any problems during the pregnancy?"
"Did you smoke, drink, or use any illicit drugs during the duration of the pregnancy?"
"Were you on any prescribed medication?"

● **B** *"Was the pregnancy full term?"*
"What was the mode of delivery?"
"Were there any complications at childbirth?"

● **C** *"Was the child breast-fed or formula-fed?"*
If formula-fed, *"What was the reason?"*
"How much and how often did you feed the child?"
If age permits, *"When and with what types of foods did the weaning process begin?"*

● **D** *"Can you tell me something about the milestones of the child?"*
or
"When did the child crawl, stand, walk, talk?"

Note: A normal child walks at 1 and talks at 2 years of age. The pincer grasp and playing the game peek-a-boo are seen at 9 months.

- **E** *"Does anyone in the house smoke?"* If no, *"Has anyone in the house ever smoked?"*
  "Does anyone in the house have any illnesses?"
  "Are there any pets in the house?"

Note: Babies in households with a known smoking history are at increased risk for sudden infant death syndrome (SIDS). Cat exposure may increase the child's risk of toxoplasmosis.

- **F** *"Have any family members or household contacts been diagnosed with any medical illnesses?"*
  "Do any of the household members currently have an upper respiratory tract infection, or any other type of transmissible disease?"
- **G** *"How is the child's growth compared to that of peers?"*

Note: It is possible that the parent may give you a growth chart to interpret at this time. You must be able to distinguish between a normal growth curve and curves indicating constitutional growth delay, short stature, or tall stature.

- **H** *"Has the child ever been hospitalized for any past medical or surgical illness?"*
- **I** *"Is the child's immunization up-to-date?"*

Psychiatric History

Obtaining the psychiatric history may be a difficult task because it is quite possible that the SP will be noncompliant. The SP may act angry to challenge you. As a rule of thumb, the best way to tackle the history is by remaining calm, polite, and assertive. Make sure that you stick to your point and assess the HPI. You may be presented with the task of completing the Mini-Mental Status exam. In this situation, you would be expected to complete this task in the given 15-minute period.

In addition to the HPI and PMH you are also required to assess the following, according to the mnemonic CASE THIS IF MORPHINE JOKE:

- **C** *"Subtract serial 3s from the number 20."*
  or
  "Spell the word 'world' backward."
- **A** Judgment of the appearance of the SP may be subjective. Make sure that you observe the SP's posture, hygiene, and any abnormal gestures.
- **S** *"Have you ever thought about killing yourself?"*
  "Have you ever thought about killing anyone else?"
- **E** *"Are you active throughout the day?"*
  or
  "Do you still have the same amount of energy as you used to?"

- **T** *"Mr./Ms. (last name), do you know where you are?"*
  "Do you know what city you are in?"
  "Do you know what year/day/month it is?"
  "Do you know who I am?"
  "Do you know what time it is?"
- **H** *"Do you hear or see things that others don't?"*
  If yes:
  "Can you describe those things to me in detail?"
- **I** *"What do you do for enjoyment?"*

- **S** This aspect can be assessed when the SP is speaking to you. The speech may be either normal or pressured, depending on how the SP presents to you.

- **I** You must look in depth at the SP's thought process to assess level of function.
- **F** *"Are you currently employed?"*
  "How is your relationship with the rest of your family?"

- **M** *"Can you tell me your date of birth, Social Security number, or wedding anniversary?"*
- **O** *"When you look at a half glass of water, do you say that the glass is half full or half empty?"*
  or
  "What are your plans for the future?"
  or
  "Would you consider yourself as someone who looks at the better side of situations or the worse side?"
- **R** *"What do I mean when I say, 'An apple a day keeps the doctor away'?"*
- **P** *"Are you suspicious of others?"*
- **H** *"How do spend your free time?"*
- **I** *"Do you get upset at small things?"*
- **N** *"What kind of daily activities do you have?"*
- **E** *"Have you ever had an out-of-body experience?"*
  or
  "Do you feel upbeat?"

- **J** *"What would you do if the empty sign of your car's gas gauge came on?"*
- **O** *"What do you think the future holds for you?"*
- **K** *"Who is the current president of United States?"*
  "Who was the first president of the United States?"
- **E** *"How is your mood these days?"*

THE PHYSICAL EXAM

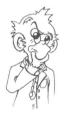

The physical exam is a significant part of the Step 2-CS exam. It should be well focused and based on the differential diagnoses. It is imperative that you perform only the pertinent and targeted physical exam in the given time period so that you will have time to complete the rest of the exam. Because you are racing the clock, no more than 5 to 7 minutes should be allotted to the focused physical exam.

The physical exam component is also scored based on a checklist filled out by the SP. Therefore, you are scored on what you are expected to do, not on what you would do in a real-life setting. The Step 2-CS emphasizes mainly the specific systems involved rather than the entire head-to-toe exam. For example, if you do a complete abdominal examination on an SP with shoulder pain, you may have wasted valuable time in which other pertinent information could have been obtained. You may have done the abdominal examination correctly, but because it was probably not on the SP's checklist, you will receive no credit for it.

THE CHECKLIST

At the end of the 15-minute SP encounter, you will leave the room to begin writing up the patient note. Meanwhile, the SP completes an assessment of the encounter. SPs are provided with a prewritten checklist that covers the questions you should have asked during the encounter. If you have covered those aspects, you will be given points for doing so. That is why it is imperative that you let the SP know exactly what you are doing. If you do not cover a certain aspect on the checklist, you will not be awarded points. If you ask questions or perform tasks that are not on the checklist, you will not be awarded points. For example, if the SP's checklist states auscultation of six areas of the chest and you auscultated eight, you will not receive extra points for the two extra areas of auscultation. You wasted valuable time that you could have used elsewhere. However, if you auscultated only four areas, you will not receive full credit either. A sample checklist for an SP complaining of pain is given below. The checklist may vary from case to case, depending on the presentation; however, the overall parameters of assessment will remain the same.

Introduction:

1. Knocked before entering?   Y   N

Did the examinee ask the following questions?
History of presenting illness:

2. Where is the location of the pain?   Y   N
3. What is the intensity of the pain on a scale of 1-10?   Y   N

19

4. What is the character of the pain?	Y	N
5. Does it radiate?	Y	N
6. Any precipitating factors?	Y	N
7. Nausea/sweating/dyspnea?	Y	N
8. Relieving and aggravating factors?	Y	N

Past medical history:

9. Any history of the HPI in the past?	Y	N
10. Any past medical or surgical illness?	Y	N
11. Any allergies to drugs or environmental factors?	Y	N

Family history:

12. Similar complaint in the family?	Y	N
13. Any medical or surgical diagnosis in the family?	Y	N

Social history:

14. Asked about alcohol use? CAGE questions?	Y	N
15. Smoking/tobacco use?	Y	N
16. Recreational drugs, IV drug use?	Y	N
17. Diet?	Y	N
18. Sexual history?	Y	N
19. Occupation?	Y	N

Physical examination:

20. Examinee washed hands before examination?	Y	N
21. Inspected the chest?	Y	N
22. Palpated for PMI?	Y	N
23. Auscultated 4 cardiac areas?	Y	N
24. Auscultated 6 areas of the lung?	Y	N
(2 anterior, 2 axillary, 2 interscapular)		

Counseling and closing:

25. Explained initial differential diagnosis in layperson's language?	Y	N
26. Described possible investigations to be done?	Y	N
27. Suggested support groups?	Y	N
28. Discussed safe sexual practices, vaccination schedule, pertinent screening exams?	Y	N

The communication skills that are addressed on the SP's checklist are graded on a scale of 1-4:

1 = Unsatisfactory, 2 = Marginally satisfactory, 3 = Good, 4 = Excellent

Communications Skills:

29. Properly introduced him- or herself?	1 2 3 4
30. Addressed SP by name?	1 2 3 4

31. Was attentive? 1 2 3 4
32. Used appropriate body language? 1 2 3 4
33. Exhibited confidence and a positive attitude? 1 2 3 4
34. Used well-mannered draping techniques? 1 2 3 4
35. Expressed empathy? 1 2 3 4
36. Asked open-ended questions? 1 2 3 4
37. Asked one question at a time? 1 2 3 4
38. Spoke clearly and understandably? 1 2 3 4
39. Acknowledged concerns and worries? 1 2 3 4
40. Verified and summarized information? 1 2 3 4
41. Used layperson's language? 1 2 3 4
42. Was well-groomed and appropriately attired? 1 2 3 4
43. Explained what he/she was doing during the physical examination? 1 2 3 4
44. Discussed various possible diagnoses? 1 2 3 4
45. Discussed various investigations? 1 2 3 4
46. Provided proper education and suggestions? 1 2 3 4
47. Was able to communicate in English? 1 2 3 4
48. Was able to correct/clarify mistakes properly? 1 2 3 4
49. Answered correctly all questions that were asked? 1 2 3 4
50. Closed case with appropriate behavior? 1 2 3 4

You must not forget the following:

1. You must tell the SP what you plan to do.
2. You must wash your hands before examining the SP.
3. You must always show compassion to the SP.
4. Comfort pain.
5. Never give water to the SP with acute abdominal pain.
6. Always auscultate before palpating an abdominal case.
7. Drape the SP when you walk in.
8. Expose only the area of the body that needs to be examined.
9. Never perform a breast, corneal, pelvic, rectal, or genital exam. If you feel that it is required for the case, you must include it in the investigation section of your SP note.
10. Never examine the SP without exposing the specific area. For example, do not auscultate over the gown.
11. Ask permission before examining the SP.
12. Warm the stethoscope before applying it to the skin surface.

Indications

SP with pain in the chest, palpitations, cough, lightheadedness, increased blood pressure, shortness of breath, diabetes mellitus, peripheral vascular disease, syncope, hematemesis, hemoptysis, pedal edema, history of myocardial infarction, angina, annual health examination.

Sequence of Examination

Inspection	Palpation	Percussion	Auscultation

Inspection

"May I untie your gown? I need to take a look at your chest."

- Look at the general appearance of the SP with open eyes for the following red flags: pallor, edema, splinter hemorrhages, marfanoid habitus, petechiae.
- After exposing the chest, look at the anterior chest wall for any abnormalities. Check for any scars, sinuses, visible pulsations, and the configuration of the rib cage.
- Identify the jugular venous pulsations. Tilt the SP to 45 degrees and with a pen torch shine light tangentially from the sternum.

Palpation

"Let me feel your heart."

- Check for any anterior chest wall tenderness.
- Palpate the radial pulses in both the upper limbs. Check for rate, rhythm, synchronicity, and volume.
- Look and palpate for the point of maximum impulse. This point is normally located at the left fifth intercostal space just internal to the midclavicular line.
- Feel for thrills in the aortic, pulmonary, tricuspid, and mitral areas.

Percussion

"May I tap your heart?"

- Percussion can be done with the respiratory examination. Many believe that percussing the cardiac borders is useless, whereas others believe that it is indicated in all cardiovascular examinations. For the Step 2-CS, it is probably not required except in cases of pericardial effusion.

Auscultation

"Let me listen to your heart. Breathe normally, please."

- Auscultate the four cardiac areas with the diaphragm of the stethoscope. Do not forget to listen to the base of the heart with the SP leaning forward.
- Also, auscultate for any carotid bruit. Then continue to palpate the carotid arteries one at a time.

RESPIRATORY SYSTEM EXAMINATION

Indications

Cough, shortness of breath, wheezing, a history of smoking, hemoptysis, hematemesis, occupational exposure (e.g., to asbestos, silicon, gravel and sand, sawdust), trauma to the chest wall, any cardiovascular case, cyanosis, clubbing, pedal edema, heartburn, annual physical examination.

Sequence of Examination

Inspection ⟶ Palpation ⟶ Percussion ⟶ Auscultation

Inspection

"May I untie your gown? I need to take a look at your chest."

- After exposing the chest wall, look for any chest wall abnormalities such as intercostal retractions, scars, bruises, and so on. Make sure that you evaluate the anterior chest wall, posterior chest wall, both axillary areas, and both supraclavicular areas.
- Evaluate the respiratory rate and pattern without the SP's knowledge to ascertain whether the SP is in any respiratory distress.
- Look for any tracheal deviation.

Palpation

"Let me feel your chest."

- Confirm any tracheal deviation with the index, middle, and ring fingers. Place the index and ring fingers on the respective sternoclavicular joint, and try to insinuate the middle finger in between them.
- Posterior chest wall expansion: Have the SP sit upright with the arms crossed in front of the chest. Place both hands, after warming, on the posterior chest wall. With the thumbs in full extension, place them parallel to the vertebral column, pinching some skin between both thumbs. Now ask the SP to take a deep breath, and look for symmetrical expansion of the chest wall.
- Tactile fremitus: With the ulnar/medial aspect of your hand placed parallel to the ribs in the intercostal space, ask the SP to repeat the phrase "ninety-nine" or "one-one-one," and feel for the vibrations transmitted to the hand. Start with the upper chest and go to the opposite side at the same level, then continue in the same fashion, alternating sides.

Percussion

"I'm now going to tap your chest. Is that alright with you?"

- Place the middle of one hand in the intercostal space, parallel to the ribs. With middle finger of the other hand (a.k.a. the pleximeter finger), strike the fixed finger. Repeat this procedure at each level, working from the top of the chest down and alternating sides, just as for chest palpation.
- Tap the axillary areas on both sides, as well as the interscapular area.
- Listen for and feel for any dullness or hyperresonance.

Auscultation

"I'm going to listen to your lungs. Breathe deeply in and out through your mouth."

- At least six areas should be auscultated with the diaphragm of the stethoscope, including both axillary areas, the apex, and the interscapular areas. Don't forget to auscultate the base of the lung. Listen for any wheezes, rales, or rhonchi. The SP may simulate these sounds.

- Warm the stethoscope before touching the chest.
- Once you have placed the diaphragm, do not move it until the SP has completed one full cycle of inspiration and expiration.

ABDOMINAL EXAMINATION

Indications

Abdominal pain, bleeding per rectum, blood-streaked stool, diarrhea, constipation, nausea, vomiting, jaundice, urinary tract infection, pregnancy, heartburn, halitosis, any obstetric/gynecology case.

Sequence of Examination

Inspection → Auscultation → Percussion → Palpation

Note: It is imperative that you auscultate prior to percussing or palpating when examining the abdomen.

Inspection

"May I lift up your gown? I need to take a look at your belly."

- After properly draping the SP from the waist downward, lift the gown upward just enough to expose the abdomen.
- Look for any scars, striae, obvious hernias, umbilicus, peristalsis, pulsations, and so on.

Auscultation

"Let me listen to your tummy."

- After warming the stethoscope, place it for 10-15 seconds anywhere on the abdomen in an attempt to hear normal/abnormal bowel sounds. Repeat at one other site.
- Listen for any renal artery bruit at a site one fingerbreadth lateral to the umbilicus on both sides.

Percussion

"I'm now going to tap your belly. If you feel any pain, please tell me."

- Place the middle of one hand on the abdomen. With the middle finger of the other hand (a.k.a. the pleximeter finger), strike the fixed finger. Tap on the four quadrants of the abdomen. Although there are nine areas, for exam purposes four will suffice.
- The normal sound on percussion is a tympanitic note, except over the liver and spleen area, where percussion will produce a dull sound.

Palpation

"I'm going to press on your belly, first lightly, then deeply. Tell me if you feel any pain."

- Light palpation: With one hand, touch the SP's abdomen in different areas lightly while observing the SP's facial expressions for any pain. Remember that the facial expression is the index of pain.
- Deep palpation: With two hands, one on top of the other, touch the SP's abdomen with a rolling motion. Palpate the area that is painful last.
- Liver palpation: Ask the SP to take a deep breath. Starting in the right lower quadrant, work your way upward to the right upper quadrant. Change hand position only after the SP expires fully.
- Spleen palpation: Ask the SP to take a deep breath. Starting in the right lower quadrant, work your way upward diagonally across to the left upper quadrant. Change hand position only after the SP expires fully.
- Check the costovertebral angle for tenderness. With the SP sitting upright, thump the area at the junction of the vertebrae and costal cartilages on both sides with a closed fist, looking for any pain associated with renal disease. An abdominal examination is never complete without this procedure.
- Rebound tenderness: In any SP presenting with an acute abdomen, this test is a necessity. On palpation the SP will feel pain when the pressure is released, not when it is applied. This test will be positive in a case of peritonitis.

CENTRAL NERVOUS SYSTEM EXAMINATION

Indications

Dizziness, vertigo, visual disturbances, weakness of the limbs, paralysis, seizures, neuropathy, headache, dementia, delirium, ataxia, tremor, poisoning, loss of consciousness.

Sequence of Examination

Mental Status ➝ Cranial Nerve ➝ Motor ➝ Reflexes ➝ Sensory ➝ Cerebellar

Note: Mc Mr Sc is the mnemonic to follow.

Mental Status Exam

- Assess the level of consciousness:

  1. Is the SP alert? Are the eyes open or closed? Does the SP look drowsy?
  2. Evaluate the SP's orientation to person, place, and time.
  3. Does the SP respond to voice or pain?

- Concentration: Have the SP spell the word *phone* backward.
- Repetition of phrases: Have the SP repeat, "Today is a sunny day."
- Memory:

  1. Short-term: Tell the SP three words, such as *apple, coffee,* and *barn.* Have the SP repeat these words later in the examination.

2. Long-term: Have the SP recall his or her date of birth, Social Security number, or wedding anniversary.

- Comprehension of written language.
- Abstraction: Does the SP understand what is meant by the saying, "An apple a day keeps the doctor away"?
- Cognitive: Have the SP name the most recent and the first president.

Cranial Nerves

- CN I (olfactory): usually omitted.
- CN II (optic):

  1. Finger count test
  2. Snellen chart for visual acuity
  3. Visual field by confrontation
  4. Direct and consensual light reflex
  5. With an ophthalmoscope, check for papilledema, retinal hemorrhages, and optic atrophy.

- CN III, IV, VI (oculomotor, trochlear, and abducent, respectively), LR-6, SO-4, O-3:

  1. Remember: A test of CN III tests all of the extraocular muscles except for the superior oblique (supplied by CN IV) and the lateral rectus (supplied by CN VI).
  2. With the SP sitting 2 feet in front of you, have the SP follow your index finger as you move it through the six cardinal positions of gaze.

- CN V (trigeminal):

  1. Motor: Ask the SP to clench the teeth, and assess the temporalis and masseter muscles as they lift the mandible.
  2. Sensory: Have the SP close both eyes and indicate when you touch the face with a cotton wisp. You must include all three divisions of the trigeminal nerve: ophthalmic, maxillary, and mandibular branches.

- CN VII (facial): Look for any signs of facial droop. Have the SP raise both eyebrows, tightly close both eyes, smile, and blow out the cheeks. Look for any facial asymmetry.
- CN VIII (vestibulocochlear): Grossly test for hearing by rubbing fingers in front of each ear. If the results are abnormal, consider performing the Rinne or Weber test.
- CN IX and CN X (glossopharyngeal and vagal, respectively): Have the SP say "aah" with a tongue depressor in place. Use a light to look for elevation of the soft palate. After asking the SP to swallow, observe for any difficulty in swallowing.
- CN XI (spinal accessory): Have the SP shrug both shoulders and turn the head from side to side against resistance.
- CN XII (hypoglossal): Have the SP protrude the tongue outside the oral cavity and move it from side to side.

Motor Assessment

- Observe! Does the SP have any atrophy or any abnormal posture or movement?
- Ask the SP to open the eyes, to look for localized findings.
- Muscle tone: Check the tone in all four extremities by asking the SP to flex and extend all four limbs.
- Muscle strength: Check by repeating the same as above, but with resistance.

1. Grade strength from 0 to 5:

   - 0 = no muscle contraction detected
   - 1 = no movement, but contraction of muscle may be evident
   - 2 = active movement with gravity
   - 3 = active movement against gravity
   - 4 = active movement against some resistance
   - 5 = active movement against full resistance

2. Upper limbs:

   - Have the SP flex the elbow (*"Please pull in"*).
   - Continue by having the SP extend the elbow (*"Push out"*).
   - Ask the SP to squeeze your fingers.

3. Lower limbs:

   - Check for hip abduction and adduction.
   - Have the SP extend and flex the knee (*"Please kick out, kick in"*).
   - Raise the SP's ankle up and down (*"Push the pedal, and release"*).

Reflexes

Deep Tendon Reflexes

- After positioning the SP properly, have him or her relax. Use a striking hammer to check the reflexes, alternating from side to side for comparison.
- You must include the biceps tendon reflex, triceps tendon reflex, and supinator, ankle, and patellar reflexes.
- For all reflexes, watch for clonus and record the briskness:

  - Grade 0 = areflexia
  - Grade 1 = weak reflex
  - Grade 2 = normal
  - Grade 3 = exaggerated
  - Grade 4 = clonus

Superficial Reflex

- With the pointed tip of your striking hammer, stroke the SP's abdomen in a diagonal fashion, watching for contraction of the abdominal muscles.

Pathological Reflex

- The Babinski reflex is elicited in individuals with an upper motor neuron lesion. Stroking the lateral aspect of the foot with the pointed tip of the striking hammer normally leads to plantar flexion. If dorsiflexion occurs, Babinski's sign is positive.

Sensory Assessment

- Explain the test to the SP before performing it.
- With the SP's eyes closed, check the pain sensation with a toothpick for pinpoint sharp pain sensation and with a wisp of cotton for light touch. Inform the SP, *"This is the pinpoint sharp pain test. Now close your eyes and indicate to me when you feel this sensation."* Do the same with the wisp of cotton.

- Test the following areas: shoulders, forearms, hand, front of thighs, calves, and feet. Remember to alternate from side to side for comparison.
- Position sense: Move the SP's finger up and down. Repeat with the other hand. Continue with the big toe of both feet. Ask the SP to identify the direction of movement.
- Vibration sense: Touch the vibrating tuning fork over the SP's distal interphalangeal joints, elbows, big toes, and medial malleolus. Have the SP indicate whether he or she can feel the vibration.

Cerebellar Assessment

- Coordination: Have the SP rapidly alternate between pronation and supination.
- Finger-to-nose test: Have the SP touch your finger and then his or her own nose.
- Heel-to-knee test: With the SP lying supine, have the SP touch the knee of one leg with the heel of the other leg and bring the heel down to the foot while not removing the heel from the leg.

HEAD/EYES/EARS/NOSE/THROAT (HEENT) EXAMINATION

Indications

Headache, head trauma, visual disturbances, tinnitus, vertigo, dizziness, sinusitis, hoarseness, epistaxis, jaw claudication, sore throat, fever, cough, jaundice, hyper- or hypothyroidism, otitis media, hearing loss, swelling in the neck, conjunctivitis, nasal discharge, halitosis, child abuse, elderly abuse, domestic violence, annual physical examination.

Head

"Let me take a look and feel your head."

- Inspect for any obvious signs of trauma, and palpate for point tenderness.
- Feel for any sinus tenderness.

Eyes

"I'm now going to look into your eyes."

- Look for any discoloration of the sclera and any conjunctival injections.
- Look at the pupils for shape, symmetry, and reactivity.
- Perform an ophthalmoscopic exam. It is necessary that you differentiate between an ophthalmoscope and an otoscope. Use your right eye for the SP's right eye, and hold the ophthalmoscope in your right hand. Repeat on the opposite side with the other eye.

Ears

"I need to pull at your ears now."

- Look for any abnormalities of the pinna. Make a note of any redness, discharge, or swelling.
- Palpate the external ear. Include the mastoid area as well.

- Perform an otoscopic exam. Remember to use a new speculum.
- The proper technique for straightening the auditory canal is to pull the pinna upward, outward, and backward.

Nose

"Let me check your nose."

- After inspecting the exterior of the nose, lift the tip of the nose and inspect the nasal turbinates with a penlight or otoscope.

Throat

"Open your mouth, stick out your tongue, and say 'aah.' "

- Inspect for tonsillar enlargement, exudates, vesicles, and dental hygiene.
- Make sure that you inspect the roof and floor of the oral cavity, as well as the buccal areas.
- You may use a tongue depressor and a penlight or otoscope if needed.
- Examine the exterior neck for scars, swelling, draining sinuses, enlargement of the thyroid, or lymphadenopathy.
- When examining the thyroid, tell the SP that you are examining the gland in the neck.
- Ask the SP to swallow, and look for normal movement of the thyroid gland.
- Palpate the gland, feeling for any enlargement, cystic or nodular. Note the temperature and fixity of the overlying skin.

MUSCULOSKELETAL SYSTEM EXAMINATION

Indications

Any joint pain, joint swelling, joint stiffness, weakness, or deformity. Shoulder pain, knee pain, and back pain are most common.

Special Tests

Sign/Test	Indicated Suspicion of
1. Obturator sign	Acute appendicitis
2. Psoas sign	Acute appendicitis
3. Kernig's sign	Suspected meningitis
4. Brudzinski's sign	Suspected meningitis
5. Murphy's sign	Acute cholecystitis
6. Tinel's sign	Carpal tunnel syndrome
7. Phalen's test	Carpal tunnel syndrome
8. Homan's sign	Deep vein thrombosis
9. Moses sign	Deep vein thrombosis
10. Anterior drawer sign	Anterior cruciate ligament tear
11. Posterior drawer sign	Posterior cruciate ligament tear
12. Weber's test	Deafness/CN VIII
13. Rinne's test	Deafness/CN VIII
14. Transillumination test	Sinusitis
15. Asterexis	Liver cell failure/hepatic encephalopathy
16. Straight leg raising test	Vertebral disc prolapse/back pain

- Inspect the area involved. If it is a bilateral joint, you must compare it with the normal side. Look for swelling, deformity, scars, sinuses, or trauma.
- Palpate the area involved and compare it with the normal side. Assess range of motion with and without resistance. Note any crepitus that may be present.
- Sensation and strength of the affected area in comparison with the normal side should also be tested.

You must know:

- Different types of gaits:

  1. Parkinson's disease: shuffling gait/festinant gait
  2. Cerebellar ataxia: broad-based gait
  3. Spastic hemiparesis: scissors gait
  4. Peripheral nerve weakness: steppage gait

- Growth charts: see Appendix
- Vaccination schedule: see Appendix
- Normal annual screening exam: see Appendix

COUNSELING, TACKLING DIFFICULT SITUATIONS, COMMUNICATING BAD NEWS

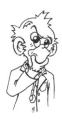

As a responsible physician, you are expected to counsel the SP regarding many aspects of patient well-being. You should address topics pertaining not only to the chief complaints but also to general overall health. For example, if the SP has a history of smoking, you are expected to discuss the negative effects of smoking. You must counsel the SP to quit smoking.

You are also required to educate the SP about screening modalities. Depending on the SP's age and family history, screening tests such as the Pap smear for cervical carcinoma, mammography for breast carcinoma, and colonoscopy for colon carcinoma should be discussed.

A discussion of diet is an integral part of counseling the SP. For example, if the SP is a diabetic, diet control is first-line management. Therefore, you are required to bring up certain issues about the benefits of maintaining a proper diet. The American Diabetic Association diet, a high-fiber diet, a low-calorie diet, or a low-sodium diet can be suggested.

The SP who has recently traveled or who plans to travel should be informed about the health risks endemic to that particular area of the world. He or she should be informed about immunization schedules, as well as possible prophylaxis.

Counseling should cover any information pertinent to the specific encounter. Depending on the situation, you might find yourself discussing any of the following with the SP:

- Alcoholics Anonymous for alcohol abuse
- Genetic counseling for congenital anomalies
- HIV testing for high-risk groups
- Possible HIV support groups for HIV-positive SPs
- Seat belt use, child car seats
- Prevention of SIDS by placing the infant on its back, avoiding stuffed toys and fluffy bedding, and cessation of smoking

- Use of smoke detectors and carbon monoxide detectors in the home
- Lead screening for high-risk groups
- The administration of folate to all women of reproductive age for the prevention of neural tube defects
- Keeping chemicals and drugs out of the reach of children
- Supervision of children in bathtubs and swimming pools
- Routine health maintenance checkups for individuals with diabetes, hypertension, and hypercholesterolemia
- Comforting the SP in distress
- Oral rehydration therapy for dehydration
- The importance of medication compliance and medication schedule adherence, as well as side effects
- Relaxation techniques such as meditation, exercise, and lifestyle changes

CHALLENGING ASPECTS OF THE SP ENCOUNTER

What if the SP keeps on talking?

It is important to understand the interview dynamic. The SP is the "boss." You must listen carefully to the information provided by the SP in order to come up with the differential diagnoses, then advise the SP about the management protocol. At the same time, the SP cannot be allowed to derail the encounter. For example, some SPs may simply talk too much. You cannot just listen casually, because you face a time constraint. The SP may intentionally try to occupy the entire session with useless gibberish. In this situation, you must tactfully interrupt the SP and continue with the encounter, according to what you need to get done. Remember to be polite. You may politely intervene by saying:

"Mr./Ms. XYZ, I know that these things have been bothering you. I fully understand your situation and will try to help you. But you have to cooperate with me and answer the questions I'm going to ask. Is that OK with you?"

Be creative. SPs have seen it all. Therefore, remember not to be rigid in regard to the questionnaire and mnemonics given in the history-taking chapter. You must be able to adapt to the encounter as needed. It is possible for the examinee not to perform well because of rigid adherence to a preset list of questions. Be flexible. Also, try to be more interactive with the SP. You should not feel that your encounter is a question-and-answer session; in actuality it is a model real-life case. If SPs came to the clinic only to answer a few questions, they could just as easily have done so by checking off boxes on a computerized questionnaire. It is your duty to "spice up" the SP encounter. Be a human first, then a doctor, and always be patient with the SP.

What if you don't know how to respond?

During the encounter the SP may ask you questions related to just about anything. Questions may be related to the SP's medical illnesses or anything else that could confuse you. SPs are doing this for a reason. It is their job to see how you will react and respond to a given situation. It is fair game for them to ask anything. Remember, in real life patients may want information about any subject, whether or not it is medically related. It is your duty to provide information that is in your specialty. SPs may ask you any of the following:

- "Doc, do I have cancer?"
- "Am I dying?"
- "Will my child be mentally retarded?"
- "Can I go on my cruise?"
- "Will I die from HIV?"
- "Am I having a heart attack?"
- "Is my chest pain just heartburn?"

Honestly, the question doesn't matter, because the answer is the same: because the SP is seeing you for the first time, you have no idea about the diagnosis or prognosis of the condition. The response to any of the above questions should be:

"*Mr./Ms. XYZ* (SP's last name), *it is very early for me to tell you what you have or what your chances are. However, I am going to complete my interview and run a couple of tests. After the results are in, we'll sit down and discuss your condition at that time. Alright? Is there anything else that you would like to ask me?*"

Leaving the ball in the SP's court is the way to go. Let the SP know that he or she is in charge. Show that you will try your level best to help the SP but that you have to understand the situation first.

Sometimes the SP may make comments such as:

- "I wish I were dead."
- "I wish I had the nerve to kill myself."
- "I wish I could die in my sleep."
- "If it weren't for my kids, my husband, I would commit suicide."
- "I hate life."
- "Why do I bother?"
- "I can't take it anymore."

All of these statements indicate suicidal intent and must be addressed immediately.

OTHER CASE FORMATS

One type of patient encounter may involve interaction with a caregiver by telephone. You may enter the room to hear the telephone ringing. Pick up the phone and say, "Hello, good morning I am Dr. XYZ in the emergency department. What can I do for you?" Be polite, listen to the voice patiently, and answer the questions appropriately. Reassure the patient or caregiver and explore the possibility of a meeting as soon as possible. If the patient says that he or she cannot come to the clinic, a physical exam is obviously not possible and will not be required. You will be provided with necessary information and instructions and will be able to take a history and ask questions. As with other cases, you will write a patient note after the encounter.

A telephone conversation/interview is an integral part of building a good doctor-patient relationship, and the art must be mastered. Even in a real-life setting there may be times when only a telephone interview is possible. For example, this technique was used during the outbreak of severe acute respiratory syndrome (SARS), when doctors themselves were dying and resorted solely to the telephone history, seeing the patient through a glass door.

Synthetic mannequins or models may be provided for assessment of sensitive exam skills involving the breast, rectum, or genital areas. In all such cases instructions will be provided.

Sometimes the SP may also show you the result of a test, an x-ray, or MRI, and ask you a challenging question.

COMMUNICATING BAD NEWS

One of the most difficult situations, even for the most experienced clinicians, is delivering unwanted information. You must tell the SP the truth. Never mislead the SP about the diagnosis and prognosis of a condition. This may be a total reversal of conceptual structures and belief systems prevalent in other parts of the world, in which the physician hides information from people with fatal illnesses and reassures them. In the United States, this practice cannot be followed. It is tantamount to malpractice.

Physicians face a lot of obstacles in this scenario. Therefore, before saying anything, you must first set the stage. You can start out by saying, *"I'm sorry, Mr./Ms. ABC, I have some bad news to tell you. I know that it is a hard time in your life. This is not easy."* Observe the SP's response, and continue. *"We just received the results of your test."* Pause, and, if possible, reach out and place your hand on the SP's shoulder or hand, then proceed. *"As we feared, the [HIV] test came back positive."* Give the SP some time to cry or deny.

The SP may now undergo any of the Kübler-Ross stages of dying: denial, anger, bargaining, depression/bereavement, or acceptance. These stages may occur in any order. You may then reach out firmly and give the SP a hug or a tissue, depending on the situation. Then give the SP some assurance. *"No matter what happens, I'll do my best to see you through this."* Show support: *"I won't abandon you, but you and I have to work together."*

CLOSING THE ENCOUNTER

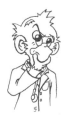

6

The last impression is a lasting impression—and you want to leave your patient with a good impression. The importance of closing cannot be overestimated, because the next step for the SP is to mark the checklist, which eventually decides the result of your encounter.

In your own words, avoiding medical terminology, summarize the important aspects of the discussion and the red flags that you may have elicited in your session with the SP. Then let the SP know what you are thinking about his or her condition and what investigations you need to perform to rule out various possibilities in the differential diagnosis. Do not scare the SP, but at the same time do not lie. Simply state plainly what you are considering in this situation. Provide comfort and reassurance. Indicate that at the next meeting the results of the investigations will be available, or schedule the next meeting as dictated by the patient's requirements. For example:

"Mr./Ms. ABC (last name preferable), *you told me that you had* ____ *and* ____. *Is that right? Now, let me sit down with you and discuss your condition. Because of what you told me, I have come up with a list of possible diagnoses. You may have* ____ *because you told me* ____. *Or you may have* ____ *because you told me* ____. *I am also thinking of the possibility that you may have* ____. *But again, it's too early to decide. I'm going to perform* ____ *to rule out/confirm* ____ *and* ____ *to rule out/confirm* ____. *If you have any questions at this time, feel free to ask me.*"

Answer the questions, but suppose that the SP has no questions. Then:

"*Well, thank you for your cooperation Mr./Ms. ABC. It was nice meeting you, and I'll call you back when the results are in. Take care, and bye for now*" (shake hands with the SP and leave the room).

7

THE PATIENT NOTE

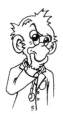

A challenging and important aspect of the Step 2-CS is writing up the patient note. It is the only documentation that you provide for a specific encounter. It basically assesses your ability to communicate findings for a particular patient to a colleague, insurance company, or hospital. In the real-life setting it is imperative that you master the art of documentation.

Once you leave the encounter and enter the workstation area, you are required to document both positive and negative findings. You have the option to write in longhand or type the notes from your encounter. A standardized worksheet that you have to fill out will be provided to you at your workstation. If you decide to type your notes, the same format will be displayed on the computer at your workstation. For both methods, your name, identification number, and station number are prewritten on the standardized form. Regardless of which method you choose, you must continue with that format for that particular encounter. You may, however, change your method of write-up in the next encounter if you choose to do so.

Once you leave the 15-minute encounter with the patient, you are given 10 minutes to complete the patient note. At the 8-minute interval a bell will sound to indicate that 2 minutes remain. If you left the patient encounter early, you may start the write-up immediately, adding extra time to the designated 10 minutes. At the end of 10 minutes, if you have not finished, the proctors will take the unfinished patient note, and you will move on to the next encounter.

As a suggestion, the differential diagnoses (five possible diagnoses) and the list of five possible investigations should be written down as soon as you reach your workstation. Once this is done, you will have completed 50% of the patient note, and you should then have enough time to gather or recall the pertinent positive and negative findings from the encounter.

THE STEP 2-CS CHEAT SHEET

Remember that at the beginning of each encounter, scratch sheets are provided for the case. They are your "cheat sheet" for the exam. It is our recommendation that you use these sheets to your best advantage. They can be used to scribble your own notes or to jot down pertinent findings during the encounter. All of the information that you have written on your scratch paper can be transferred to the patient note. The piece of scratch paper that you use during an encounter will be collected at the end of the 10 minutes allotted to the write-up, along with your patient note. The scratch paper will be destroyed and will not change your score.

As soon as the encounter begins, before you knock on the door and after you read the information in the door box, our recommendation is to divide your scratch paper into 4 + 1 quadrants, designating a box for the HPI, PMI, list of possible diagnoses, list of possible investigations, additional questions to be asked of the patient, and counseling information (see Appendix).

Using the cheat sheet this way provides you with a clean road map before you begin the encounter. You also have the opportunity to change it as common sense and the encounter dictate. Basically, this format makes life a lot easier. Any mnemonic that you need can be easily written on the cheat sheet in the respective box. Anything that you may forget to ask the patient is also taken care of.

WRITING THE NOTE PROPER

Writing the patient note will be much easier if you follow the above format on your cheat sheet. We cannot overemphasize the importance of that cheat sheet. If it is properly completed, you have only to copy the information from the cheat sheet to your standardized patient note, thereby saving time and making life a lot easier. Because everyone has his or her own style of case presentation, it is also your choice if you want to write in paragraph format or list the appropriate information in a series of points. Thus, individuality is respected.

SAMPLE PATIENT NOTE

History

- The chief complaint should be in the SP's own words. The rest of the story can be written based on the mnemonics for the HPI and PMH.
- You must also include all negative history findings.

Physical Examination

- On the first line, the vital signs may be copied from the information provided in the box on the door, and abnormal findings may be underlined or circled.
- For the general appearance of the SP, the mnemonic PICCLE can be used:
  - **P**   Pallor
  - **I**   Icterus
  - **C**   Clubbing
  - **C**   Cyanosis
  - **L**   Lymphadenopathy
  - **E**   Edema

- Then you may make a note about how the SP presents to you. For example, "patient is conscious, cooperative, sitting comfortably on the examination table, and in no apparent distress."
- You must then list the relevant systems exam findings.
- Never use terms such as "unremarkable," "nil", or "N/A." Be specific.

Abbreviations

On the exam, common medical abbreviations can be used. Writing out everything can take up vital time. For a comprehensive list of abbreviations, see the Appendix.

MODEL CASES

Cardiovascular Examination

- Pulses 2+, B/L, regular (or diminished and irregular)
- No sinuses, scars on the chest wall
- No JVD
- PMI nondisplaced (or PMI laterally displaced)
- No palpable heaves or thrills
- S_1, S_2 +, no gallops (or prominent S_4 gallop), no added heart sounds

Respiratory Examination

- N. breathing and RR
- Trachea in the midline
- No mediastinal shift
- N. tactile fremitus, no dullness on percussion
- NVBS B/L or chest B/L clear
- No rhonchi, rales, pleural rubs, or adventitious sounds

HEENT Examination

- Head: N. cephalic, atraumatic, no point tenderness
- Eyes: no yellowish discoloration, no redness, no discharge, EOM intact, PERLA, fundus N., no papilledema or vascular changes B/L
- Ears: no tenderness, discharge B/L, TM clear, N. light reflex
- Nose: no apparent septal deviation, no discharge, nasal turbinates not congested, no polyps
- Throat: oropharynx clear, good dental hygiene, no thrush, no exudates, no tonsillar enlargement.
- Neck: supple, no cervical LN enlargement, no thyroid enlargement

Central Nervous System Examination

- Pt. alert, oriented × 3
- CN nerves II–XII intact
- Motor N strength 5/5
- Reflexes DTR 2+, no Babinski
- Intact pain and temp
- (−) Rhomberg test, finger/nose test intact

Abdominal Examination

- Abd. scaphoid, no scars, sinuses, or striae
- BS, NT/ND
- Abd. tympanitic note all quads
- Abd. soft, no organomegaly, no palpable masses
- No rebound tenderness
- No CVAT

Musculoskeletal Examination

- No obvious signs of deformity, or trauma
- No point tenderness
- ROM intact B/L
- N. sensations
- No warmth B/L

Psychiatry Examination

- Pt. appears disheveled, unkempt
- Alert and oriented × 3
- Memory recent and remote intact
- Pressured speech
- Depressed mood
- Affect consistent with mood
- Auditory or visual hallucinations
- *Suicidal ideation* (you must underline red alerts)
- No homicidal ideation
- Judgment impaired

SOME ADVICE FOR REAL LIFE

Try to practice compassion in everyday life. In professional practice, the combination of an open heart and politeness can go a long way. Knowing the stress of these board exams and the toll it can take on you, you must look and imagine beyond it. It is not the exam that will test your medical ability; it is the patient that you will cure. If you prepare for these exams with zest, zeal, and vigor, understanding what kind of change you can make in a person's life, you are already one step ahead of the game.

A kind and caring word at the right time can bring solace to the distressed patient. This definitely improves the doctor-patient relationship. This is what you want at the end of the day. This is the basis of a healthier and more productive energy that has the potential to take us to greater heights of inner satisfaction. The following pedagogical motto should be tattooed in your mind throughout your career in this "noble profession":

"He longed to soothe her, not with drugs, not with advice, but with simple kindly words."

Anton Chekhov, "A Doctor's Visit"

During all your clinical rotations, formulate your own style of history taking. Assess, reassess, and evaluate yourself. Even more important, take into consideration the evaluation of your peers and senior colleagues. Then and only then can you adapt and evolve into a better physician. It is this form of evaluation that will fill in your deficiencies, not the intellectual nourishment of the board exams.

65 Sample Cases

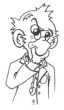

8

Case 1: Melizabeth Baylor, a 58-year-old woman with chest pain for the past 4 hours

Case 2: Justin Jimberlake, a 24-year-old man complaining of chest pain for the past 3 days

Case 3: Nack Jicholson, a 62-year-old man with back pain

Case 4: Fritney Smears, a 22-year-old woman with back pain

Case 5: Catherine Beta-Cones, a 28-year-woman with pain and swelling in the right knee

Case 6: Tanet Backson, a 34-year-old woman with pain in the shoulder

Case 7: Dudy Jench, a 66-year-old woman with pain in her knee

Case 8: Kashton Fitcher, a 23-year-old man with cough for the past 2 weeks

Case 9: Bill Bosby, a 62-year-old male smoker with cough

Case 10: Prad Bitt, an 18-year-old man with bleeding nose

Case 11: Foscar Lyle, a 26-year-old man with bleeding per rectum

Case 12: Sal Lupino, a 62-year-old man with bleeding per rectum

Case 13: Cariah Marey, a 33-year-old woman with complaints of vomiting

Case 14: Sean Sceanarry, a 62-year-old man with blurred vision

Case 15: Sally McDeal, a 32-year-old woman with palpitations

Case 16: Fichael Rox, a 65-year-old man with tremors

Case 17: Gemma Ovary, a 42-year-old woman with a malodorous vaginal discharge

Case 18: Lennifer Jopez, a 22-year-old woman with nausea, vomiting, and yellowness of the eyes

Case 19: Meddie Eurphy, a 55-year-old man with constipation

Case 20: Cameron Tiaz, a 20-year-old woman with complaints of lower abdominal pain, fever, and cervical discharge for 1 week

Case 21: Brandy Arcia, a 60-year-old man with a history of peripheral vascular disease and an ulcer on his left leg with purulent discharge

Case 22: Halma Sayek, a 30-year-old woman with loose stools

Case 23: Kanna Oournikova, a 54-year-old woman who has not seen a doctor for the past 20 years

Case 24: Armen Selectra, a 27-year-old woman with fever, headache, nausea, photophobia, and a history of sinusitis

Case 25: Gichard Rere, a 53-year-old man with fatigue, recurrent nose bleeds, and tachypnea

Case 26: Jashley Hudd, a 24-year-old woman with headache, pain in the malar area, and a tenacious green mucoid discharge

Case 27: Lennifer Hove Jewit, a 30-year-old woman with diarrhea

Case 28: Meve Startin, a 60-year-old man complaining of memory loss and progressive mental deterioration

Case 29: Ellen Unt, a 28-year-old woman with pain and tingling in the hand

Case 30: Hustin Doffman, a 70-year-old man complaining of frequent falls

Case 31: Memi Doore, a 40-year-old woman complaining of lack of energy and difficulty sleeping

Case 32: Mrs. Smith, whose 8-month-old child has fever, rash, and convulsions

Case 33: Rulia Joberts, a 40-year-old woman with weight loss for the past 3 months

Case 34: Candy Awford, a 30-year-old woman complaining of weight gain

Case 35: Brock Hudson, a 36-year-old man who was diagnosed with HIV 3 years ago

Case 36: Amela Panderson, a 52-year-old woman complaining of dyspareunia

Case 37: Tuma Hurman, the mother of a 1-week-old boy who is yellow in color

Case 38: Gel Mibson, whose 9-year-old daughter is shorter than her peers

Case 39: Tohn Javoltra, a 40-year-old man complaining of fatigue

Case 40: George Gloomy, a 42-year-old man complaining of excessive daytime sleepiness/insomnia

Case 41: Jeeter Pennings, a 52-year-old man who comes to your clinic for his health checkup

Case 42: Roxanne Starr, a 40-year-old obese woman with right upper quadrant pain, fever, and emesis

Case 43: Fristina Cingulara, a 28-year-old woman with pain in her right flank

Case 44: Annifer Janiston, a 22-year-old woman presenting to the ED with complaints of right lower abdominal pain and lack of appetite

Case 45: Evita Scleron, a 44-year-old woman complaining that she was a victim of domestic abuse

Case 46: Billy Bob Borton, a 47-year-old man complaining of bad breath

Case 47: James Dameron, a 27-year-old man complaining of hiccups

Case 48: Celine De Old, a 34-year-old woman complaining of hoarseness

Case 49: Dobert Role, a 48-year-old man complaining of impotence

Case 50: Hugh Brant, a 31-year-old man with pain on the left side of his face

Case 51: Tina Mourner, a 17-year-old girl who has never had a menstrual period

Case 52: Becky Harpe, a 37-year-old woman complaining of postcoital bleeding

Case 53: Bule Brenner, a 68-year-old male smoker complaining of difficulty swallowing solids and a 15-pound weight loss

Case 54: Kevin Jostner, a 51-year-old man with an increased urge to void urine

Case 55: Jim Marry, a 46-year-old man complaining of unsteadiness and instability

Case 56: Martha Beuhart, a 38-year-old woman who claims that she has been sexually assaulted

Case 57: Nicole Hitman, a 36-year-old woman with a history of recurrent spontaneous abortions

Case 58: Sally Feeds, a 28-year-old woman with hematemesis

Case 59: Jackie Dhan, a 36-year-old man complaining of itching

Case 60: Toby McDire, a 23-year-old man brought to the ED by paramedics after a high-speed motor vehicle accident with complaints of difficult breathing

Case 61: Adam Mandler, a 22-year-old medical student who is overly stressed by the USMLE Step 2-CS and takes 30 tablets from an unlabeled bottle

Case 62: Kate Hoss, a thin 23-year-old woman on a crash diet because she thinks she is overweight

Case 63: Melon Herren, a 27-year-old woman with a history of amenorrhea for the past 2 months and complaints of nausea and vomiting

Case 64: Russell Browe, a 32-year-old man who is brought to the clinic by his wife because he hit his neighbor and took away his neighbor's cat

Case 65: Jennifer Fairy, a 47-year-old disheveled women brought to the ED by her husband for financial extravagance

Case 1   Melizabeth Baylor is a 58-year-old woman with chest pain for the past 4 hours.

Differential Diagnoses (mnemonic: M-CAPUT)

1. Myocardial infarction
2. Carditis
3. Aortic dissection
4. Pulmonary embolism
5. Unstable angina
6. Tension pneumothorax
7. Gastroesophageal reflux disease
8. Costochondritis
9. Pneumonia
10. Trauma

Investigations

1. ECG
2. Cardiac enzymes (CPK-MB, troponin)
3. Chest x-ray
4. CBC with differential count (DC)
5. Electrolytes
6. Echocardiography
7. V/Q scan
8. Arterial blood gases
9. Barium swallow
10. EGD

Red Flags

1. Smoking, hyperlipidemia, diabetes mellitus, age, male sex, and type A personality are risk factors for myocardial infarction.
2. Pain that is worse when lying down or with a heavy meal, alcohol, or smoking strongly suggests gastroesophageal reflux disease.
3. Female sex, DVT, OCP, a history of surgery, and immobility are risk factors for pulmonary embolism.
4. Marfanoid features suggest aortic dissection.

Focused History

- Pain: Use LIQOR DRAW mnemonic
- Associated symptoms to ask about:

  ☐ Dyspnea: If present, how short of breath is the patient? When does it occur—at night or when the patient is sitting?
  ☐ Palpitations: What precipitates them? Are they regular or irregular?
  ☐ Cough history
  ☐ Edema: Does swelling occur in the feet or the face?
  ☐ Cramplike pain in calves when walking that is relieved by rest
  ☐ Coldness/blueness of extremities
  ☐ Past history of rheumatic fever

Targeted Physical Examination

- General exam
- Complete CVS and RS exams

Case 2   Justin Jimberlake is a 24-year-old man complaining of chest pain for the past 3 days.

Differential Diagnoses

1. Pneumonia
2. Mitral valve prolapse
3. Hypertrophic cardiomyopathy
4. Esophageal spasm
5. Costochondritis
6. Fractured rib
7. Gastroesophageal reflux disease
8. Perforated peptic ulcer
9. Pericarditis
10. Acute chest syndrome
11. Myocardial infarction

Investigations

1. Chest x-ray
2. Echocardiography
3. CBC with DC
4. Electrolytes
5. Barium swallow

6. EGD
7. ECG
8. CPK-MB, troponin
9. X-ray of abdomen
10. US of abdomen

Red Flags

1. Fever, cough, shortness of breath, and nausea are red flags for pneumonia.
2. Palpitation, pain, panic attack, and syncope suggest mitral valve prolapse.
3. In a patient with severe anemia, cocaine toxicity, or a history of carbon monoxide poisoning, suspect MI.
4. In an African-American patient with a history of sickle cell anemia, suspect acute chest syndrome.

Focused History

- LIQOR DRAW mnemonic for pain
- History of sickle cell disease: If present, ask about fever, dehydration, severe exertion, recent travel to high altitude, hematuria, and history of blood transfusion.

Targeted Physical Examination

- General
- Complete CVS and RS exams

Case 3   Nack Jicholson is a 62-year-old man with back pain.

Differential Diagnoses

1. Lumbar disk herniation
2. Trauma
3. Abdominal aortic aneurysm
4. Pancreatitis
5. Spinal canal stenosis
6. Metastatic deposits
7. Degenerative lumbosacral arthritis
8. Spinal cord tumor
9. Sciatica
10. Cauda equina syndrome
11. Epidural abscess

Investigations

1. CBC with DC
2. X-ray of lumbosacral spine
3. Rectal exam
4. MRI
5. CT myelogram
6. Nerve conduction study
7. Prostate-specific antigen/alkaline phosphatase levels

8. Bone scan
9. Serum amylase, lipase levels
10. Electromyogram

Red Flags

1. Sensory disturbances, lower extremity weakness, sphincter or sexual dysfunction, and, above all, pain that increases with intrathoracic pressure suggest lumbar disk herniation.
2. A history of fever, cancer, weight loss, trauma with bowel or bladder incontinence, and saddle anesthesia suggests cauda equina syndrome.
3. A history of alcohol use or gallstones suggests pancreatitis.

Focused History

- LIQOR DRAW mnemonic for pain

Targeted Physical Examination

- General exam
- Abdominal exam. Specifically palpate for a pulsatile mass (AAA) and feel for femoral pulses
- Back exam

  ☐ Inspection: erythema, contusions or previous scars
  ☐ Palpation for point tenderness
  ☐ Percussion of vertebral bodies

- Neurologic exam of lower limb
- Straight-leg-raising test
- Lasegue test (foot dorsiflexion)

Case 4   Fritney Smears is a 22-year-old woman with back pain.

Differential Diagnoses

1. Ankylosing spondylitis
2. Pelvic inflammatory disease
3. Menstrual cramps
4. Spinal stenosis
5. Hypochondriasis
6. Irritable bowel disease
7. Ulcerative colitis

Investigations

1. CBC with DC
2. Electrolytes
3. Cervical culture and smear
4. X-ray of abdomen
5. CT scan
6. MRI
7. Rectal exam
8. Pelvic exam
9. HLA B-27 testing

Red Flags

1. Family history, usually in a male patient, and morning stiffness that improves with exercise suggest ankylosing spondylitis.
2. Pain related to position (for example, a patient who can ride a bike but cannot walk) suggests spinal stenosis.

Focused History

- LIQOR DRAW mnemonic for pain

Targeted Physical Examination

- General exam
- Abdominal exam and CVAT
- Back exam

  - ☐ Inspection: erythema, contusions, or previous scars
  - ☐ Palpation for point tenderness
  - ☐ Percussion of vertebral bodies

- Neurologic exam of lower limb
- Straight-leg-raising test
- Lasegue test (foot dorsiflexion)

Case 5   Catherine Beta-Cones is 28-year-old woman with pain and swelling in the right knee.

Differential Diagnoses

1. Rheumatoid arthritis
2. Septic arthritis
3. Traumatic hemarthrosis
4. Meniscal injury (must examine both knees)
5. Fracture
6. Chondrosarcoma
7. Osteoid osteoma
8. Crystal-induced arthropathy
9. Systemic lupus erythematosus
10. Reiter's syndrome
11. Lyme disease

Investigations

1. CBC with DC
2. ESR
3. CRP
4. Plain x-ray films
5. Arthrocentesis: 3 Cs (culture, count, crystal)
6. MRI
7. Rh factor
8. ANA, anti-DS-DNA, anti-Smith antibodies
9. Bone scan

10. IgM antibody
11. Culture of blood, urethra, rectum, and cervix

 ### Red Flags

1. Conjunctivitis, urethritis, and arthritis suggest Reiter's syndrome.
2. Symmetrical arthritis suggests rheumatoid arthritis.
3. Monarticular arthritis suggests septic arthritis.
4. A bull's-eye rash and a history of a tick bite suggest Lyme disease.
5. A butterfly rash suggests systemic lupus erythematosus.
6. A petechial rash with tenosynovitis suggests gonococcal arthritis.

Focused History

- Pain history
- Any fever, nausea, or diarrhea
- History of travel and tick bite
- Any rash
- Any pain or joint swelling elsewhere in the body
- Sexual history

Targeted Physical Examination

- General exam
- Check knee for full range of motion.
- Check for effusion by ballottement.
- Check the other knee.
- Grossly check all other joints.
- Brief CVS and RS exams

Case 6   Tanet Backson is a 34-year-old woman with pain in the shoulder.

Differential Diagnoses

1. Rotator cuff tear
2. Shoulder dislocation
3. Fracture
4. Septic arthritis
5. History of electroconvulsive therapy (ECT)
6. Seizures
7. Subacromial bursitis
8. Myocardial infarction
9. Domestic violence
10. Frozen shoulder (adhesive capsulitis)

Investigations

1. X-ray of shoulder: AP, lateral, tangential, and scapular views
2. CBC with DC
3. ESR
4. Arthrocentesis

5. MRI
6. Ultrasound of shoulder
7. ECG

Red Flags

1. Trauma to the shoulder may cause fracture or dislocation.
2. A history of depression suggests possible treatment with ECT.
3. In a patient with bruises or multiple fractures with no reasonable explanation, domestic violence should be suspected.
4. Female sex, age, shoulder trauma, surgery, diabetes, and hemiplegia are associated with frozen shoulder.

Note: Don't shake hands with the patient. You may worsen the pain! Remember to examine both shoulders.

Focused History

- Pain history
- Any pain or joint swelling elsewhere in the body
- History of trauma
- Sexual history

Targeted Physical Examination

- General exam
- Check shoulder for full range of motion.
- Check the other shoulder.
- Grossly check all other joints.
- Feel for the radial and brachial pulses in the limb involved.
- Brief CVS, RS exams

Case 7   Dudy Jench is a 66-year-old woman with pain in her knee.

Differential Diagnoses

1. Degenerative arthritis
2. Infective arthritis
3. Osteoporosis
4. Trauma/fracture
5. Metastatic malignancy
6. Gout
7. Multiple myeloma
8. Drug-induced pain

Investigations

1. X-ray of knee
2. Arthrocentesis (3 Cs)
3. Blood calcium levels
4. Albumin
5. Phosphate

6. BC with DC
7. Serum uric acid levels
8. ESR
9. Bence-Jones protein
10. DEXA scan

Red Flags

1. Wear and tear of old age suggests osteoarthritis.
2. Menopause suggests osteoporosis.
3. A history of hydralazine, quinidine, corticosteroid, barbiturate, or anticoagulant use suggests drug-induced pain.

Focused History

- Pain history
- Any pain or joint swelling elsewhere in the body
- History of trauma
- Sexual history

Targeted Physical Examination

- General exam
- Check knee for full range of motion.
- Check for effusion by ballottement.
- Check the other knee.
- Grossly check all other joints.
- Brief CVS and RS exams

Case 8   Kashton Fitcher is a 23-year-old man with a cough for the past 2 weeks.

Differential Diagnoses

1. Pneumonia
2. Tuberculosis
3. Smoking
4. Asthma
5. Bronchitis
6. Allergy
7. Drug-induced cough
8. Postnasal drip due to sinusitis
9. Bronchiectasis/cystic fibrosis
10. Emphysema

Investigations

1. CBC with DC
2. Purified protein derivative test
3. Chest x-ray
4. Sputum culture and sensitivity, acid-fast stain

5. Electrolytes
6. X-ray of paranasal sinuses
7. Sweat chloride test

Red Flags

1. Fever suggests pneumonia.
2. History of smoking (very important).
3. Use of ACE inhibitors or beta-blockers suggests drug-induced cough.
4. History of allergy.

Focused History

- Cough: onset, duration, aggravating and relieving factors, dry or productive, color and quantity of sputum if productive
- Associated breathing problems, chest pain, or any pain of pleuritic nature; fever and exposure history, travel history, smoking history

Targeted Physical Examination

- General exam
- Complete RS exam
- CVS exam

Case 9

Bill Bosby is a 62-year-old male smoker with a cough.

Differential Diagnoses

1. Bronchogenic carcinoma
2. Chronic bronchitis
3. Congestive cardiac failure
4. Tuberculosis
5. Pneumonia
6. Aspiration
7. Medications
8. Bronchiectasis

Investigations

1. Chest x-ray
2. CT of chest
3. Sputum cytology
4. CBC with DC
5. Electrolytes
6. Bronchoscopy
7. Thoracoscopy
8. Mediastinoscopy
9. MRI brain for metastasis
10. Purified protein derivative test

Red Flags

1. A smoking history, asbestosis, and silicosis (from occupational exposure), with hemoptysis: the odds overwhelmingly favor lung cancer.
2. Alcoholism suggests aspiration.

Focused History

- Cough history, associated history, smoking history
- Occupational history:

    □ Is the job dusty? If so, what tools make the dust?
    □ Are dangerous or toxic fumes or vapors involved?
    □ What kind of protection is used?
    □ Has any similar illness affected another employee?

Targeted Physical Examination

- General exam
- Complete RS and brief CVS exam
- Examination of lymph nodes

Case 10   Prad Bitt is an 18-year-old man with a bleeding nose.

Differential Diagnoses

1. Trauma
2. Juvenile nasopharyngeal angiofibroma (JNA)
3. Coagulopathy (hemophilia A or B, idiopathic thrombocytopenic purpura, von Willebrand's disease)
4. Leukemia
5. Foreign body
6. Fracture nasal bone
7. Drug-induced reaction
8. Vitamin K or C deficiency

Investigations

1. CBC with DC
2. Prothrombin time, partial thromboplastin time (PT/PTT)
3. Bleeding time/clotting time
4. Rhinoscopy
5. Bone marrow biopsy
6. CT scan
7. Platelet count
8. Ristocetin test
9. Factor VIII assay
10. Mixing study

Red Flags

1. A history of repeated nose picking suggests trauma.
2. A history of anticoagulant, aspirin, or cytotoxic drug use suggests drug-induced bleeding.

3. Platelet bleeding suggests a superficial type of bleeding.
4. Factor bleeding suggests a deep type of bleeding.
5. JNA presents with profuse epistaxis in a boy near puberty.

Focused History

- History of trauma/repeated digital nose picking, foreign body trauma or attempts at removal
- Associated bleeding disorders
- Fever, headache, nasal obstruction
- History of drug use (e.g., anticoagulants)
- History of travel

Targeted Physical Examination

- General exam
- Inspection of nose, palpation of nose and paranasal sinuses (may elicit tenderness)
- Forward bending test and transillumination test
- Brief CVS and RS exams

Case 11 Foscar Lyle is a 26-year-old man with bleeding per rectum.

Differential Diagnoses

1. Hemorrhoids (most common cause in the young)
2. Angiodysplasia
3. Infectious disease
4. Inflammatory bowel disease
5. Meckel's diverticulum
6. Colon cancer
7. Anal intercourse
8. Drug-induced bleeding
9. Gastric ulcer/duodenal ulcer
10. Variceal bleeding

Investigations

1. Rectal exam
2. Orthostatic vital signs
3. Fecal occult blood test
4. Anoscopy, sigmoidoscopy, colonoscopy
5. Bleeding scan
6. Nasogastric lavage
7. CBC with DC
8. Endoscopy

Red Flags

1. Hematochezia is bright red blood passed per rectum. Melena is black tarry stools.
2. Orthostatic hypotension indicates greater than 20% blood loss.
3. Extraintestinal manifestations occur in inflammatory bowel disease.

Case 12   Sal Lupino is a 62-year-old man with bleeding per rectum.

Differential Diagnoses

1. Carcinoma of the colon
2. Diverticular bleeding
3. Anal fissure
4. Mesenteric ischemia
5. Drug-induced bleeding
6. Polyps
7. Inflammatory bowel disease
8. Intussusception
9. Trauma

Investigations

1. Rectal exam
2. Orthostatic vital signs
3. Fecal occult blood test
4. Anoscopy, sigmoidoscopy, colonoscopy
5. BUN, creatinine levels
6. Bleeding scan
7. Nasogastric lavage
8. CBC with DC
9. Endoscopy

Red Flags

1. In an elderly patient, abdominal pain out of proportion to findings on the physical exam and bleeding per rectum suggest mesenteric ischemia.
2. Loss of weight, loss of appetite, and caliber of stools in an elderly patient suggest colon cancer. The right side bleeds and the left side obstructs.

Case 13   Cariah Marey is a 33-year-old woman with complaints of vomiting.

Differential Diagnoses

1. Pregnancy
2. Food poisoning
3. Cholecystitis
4. Appendicitis
5. Migraine
6. Motion sickness
7. Labyrinthitis
8. Bulimia/anorexia nervosa
9. Drug-induced vomiting
10. Hepatitis

Investigations

1. Pregnancy test
2. CBC with DC
3. Electrolytes
4. BUN, creatinine levels
5. AST, ALT, alkaline phosphatase
6. US of abdomen
7. CT scan of abdomen
8. X-rays of abdomen, acute series

Red Flags

1. Amenorrhea, breast tenderness, and so on suggest the morning sickness complex of pregnancy.
2. Trigger factors that cause the headache indicate migraine.
3. Use of aspirin, estrogen, chemotherapy, digoxin, metronidazole, or ipecac, as well as the use of any drug, can cause vomiting and nausea.

Focused History

- Ask about onset and nature of vomiting, fever, abdominal pain, vaginal bleeding, headache.
- Obtain a complete obstetric/gynecologic history.
- Ask about rubella immunization.

Targeted Physical Examination

- General exam
- Abdominal exam
- Brief CVS, RS exams
- Examination of lower limb for edema/varicose veins

Case 14   Sean Sceanarry is a 62-year-old man with blurred vision.

Differential Diagnoses

1. Cataract
2. Glaucoma
3. Myopia/hypermetropia
4. Retinal detachment
5. Optic neuritis
6. Transient ischemic attack/cerebrovascular accident
7. Migraine
8. Temporal arteritis
9. Multiple sclerosis
10. Central retinal vein or artery occlusion (CRVO, CRAO)
11. Macular degeneration
12. Hypertensive retinopathy
13. Diabetic retinopathy
14. Trauma
15. Conjunctivitis

Investigations

1. Visual acuity/visual fields
2. Tonometry
3. Blood sugar/hemoglobin 1ac
4. Carotid artery Doppler
5. Biopsy of temporal artery
6. ESR
7. CBC with DC

Red Flags

1. Sudden, painful loss of vision suggests trauma, optic neuritis, migraine, or glaucoma.
2. Sudden, painless loss of vision suggests CRVO, CRAO, retinal detachment, transient ischemic attack, or cerebrovascular accident.
3. Gradual loss of vision suggests cataract, diabetic retinopathy, presbyopia, or other refractive errors.

Focused History

- Onset, progression, and duration of blurred vision
- Any other sensory changes, vertigo, and so on
- History of diabetes mellitus, hypertension

Targeted Physical Examination

- General exam
- Ophthalmoscopic exam
- Brief neurologic exam of sensory system
- Check vibration and position sense
- Auscultate carotid arteries
- Brief CVS

Case 15 Sally Mc Deal is a 32-year-old woman with palpitations.

Differential Diagnoses

1. Panic disorder with/without agoraphobia
2. Hyperthyroidism
3. Mitral valve prolapse
4. Supraventricular tachycardia
5. Generalized anxiety disorder
6. Substance abuse
7. Hypoglycemia
8. Pheochromocytoma
9. Drug-induced palpitations

Investigations

1. ECG
2. T_3, T_4, thyroid-stimulating hormone (TSH)
3. CBC with DC

4. Electrolytes
5. Urine and serum toxicology screen
6. Blood glucose
7. Urine vanillylmandelic acid

Red Flags

1. Fear or trouble on leaving home, suicidal ideation, and hallucinations suggest panic disorder.
2. Episodic hypertension and headache suggest pheochromocytoma.

Focused History

- When did this awareness of an irregular heartbeat begin?
- What precipitates the palpitations?
- How long do they last?
- Do they have any relationship to exercise or stress?
- Does the heart give an occasional thump?
- Do they have any relationship to pulse?
- Has the patient had dyspnea, pain, or syncopal attacks?

Targeted Physical Examination

- General exam
- Complete CVS, brief RS
- Thyroid examination

Case 16 Fichael Rox is a 65-year-old man with tremors.

Differential Diagnoses

1. Senile tremors
2. Hyperthyroidism
3. Hypoglycemia
4. Alcohol withdrawal
5. Benign essential tremors
6. Parkinson's disease
7. Increased caffeine use
8. Medication
9. Hepatic failure
10. Electrolyte imbalance

Investigations

1. CBC with DC
2. Electrolytes
3. T_3, T_4, TSH levels
4. Blood sugar
5. Toxicology screen
6. BUN, creatinine levels
7. AST, ALT, alkaline phosphatase

8. CT or MRI of head
9. CT of abdomen
10. Insulin, C-peptide levels

Red Flags

1. The tremor should be classified as to body part (arms, head), activation condition (when the tremor is present), frequency (fast or slow), and amplitude (fine or coarse).
2. Tremor and rigidity may become more pronounced if the patient performs voluntary movements with the opposite limb (e.g., the patient draws a circle in the air with the opposite hand). The patient is asked to stand and to walk, thus revealing any evidence of difficulty initiating movement, reduced arm swing, or shuffling gait.
3. If the tremor is caused by stroke, the onset is usually acute, and the patient may appear ill and complain of headache, vertigo, and difficulty with balance. Observe for nystagmus, difficulty with speech or swallowing, and uneven gait (falling to one side).
4. Multiple sclerosis is suspected if the tremor is associated with visual disturbances and diverse neurologic symptoms and signs.
5. Check for evidence of chronic alcoholism, including spider angiomas, gynecomastia, enlarged liver, or abnormal blood test results (elevated mean corpuscular volume or gamma-glutamyltransferase [GGT] level).
6. If weight loss, irritability, a racing heart, or neck swelling is described, the patient should be examined for thyroid enlargement, exophthalmos, brisk reflexes, and tachycardia.
7. Tremor occurring 3–4 hours after eating may suggest hypoglycemia. Other signs of hypoglycemia include altered sensorium, sweating, and pallor.
8. Tremor in conjunction with feelings of suffocation, chest tightness, and a racing heart may indicate panic disorder.
9. Hand tremor, sleep disturbance, irritability, sweating, nausea, and difficulty with concentration may indicate benzodiazepine withdrawal. The physician should ask about the patient's use of prescription or over-the-counter medications that are known to cause tremor.
10. Use of epinephrine, isoprotenerol, theophylline, caffeine, lithium, thyroid hormones, tricyclic antidepressants, or valproic acid may cause drug-induced tremors.
11. The combination of tremors, rigidity, bradykinesia, and postural instability suggests Parkinson's disease.
12. Increased insulin and hypoglycemia that improve after the patient eats constitute Whipple's triad.
13. Essential tremor is a possibility if the examination is normal except for postural tremor and a positive family history.
14. Anxiety or nervousness causes fine tremors or physiologic tremors (the most common cause).

Focused History

■ Determine onset, exacerbating and relieving factors, medications, family history, and associated symptoms
■ Assess functional limitations, including job-related disabilities, social embarrassment, and difficulty with holding a cup or handwriting

Targeted Physical Examination

1. General exam: Observation is the initial step in the physical exam. Observe the patient sitting with the hands resting in the lap or standing with the arms at the sides. Look for exophthal-

mos (thyrotoxicosis), a flushed face (alcoholism), a masklike face (parkinsonism), an anxious face (anxiety), very old age (senile tremors, parkinsonism).

2. Ask the patient to extend the arms and perform the finger-to-nose or finger-to-finger movement to identify an intention tremor. Observe the patient drinking from a glass, writing, or drawing a rhythmic pattern such as a spiral.

3. In a patient with resting tremor, check for rigidity and bradykinesia by flexing and extending the patient's arms, seeking signs of cogwheel rigidity.

4. Perform brief CNS, CVS, and RS exams.

5. Perform a thyroid exam.

6. Ask the patient to protrude the tongue to check for fasciculation.

7. Make a note of head nodding if present.

8. If intention tremor is present, do a cerebellar function test.

Case 17   Gemma Ovary is a 42-year-old woman with a malodorous vaginal discharge.

Differential Diagnoses

1. Bacterial vaginosis
2. Candidiasis
3. Trichomoniasis
4. Gonorrhea
5. Chlamydial infection
6. Foreign body
7. Poor hygiene

Investigations

1. Pelvic exam
2. Wet mount
3. KOH preparation
4. pH of vaginal fluid
5. Whiff test
6. Urine analysis
7. USG of abdomen
8. Culture with Nickerson's medium for candidiasis

Red Flags

1. Pregnancy, diabetes mellitus, broad-spectrum antibiotics, corticosteroids, heat, moisture, and occlusive clothing predispose to candidiasis.
2. Both partners must be treated for trichomoniasis.

Case 18 Lennifer Jopez is a 22-year-old woman with nausea, vomiting, and yellowness of the eyes.

Differential Diagnoses

1. Viral hepatitis
2. Alcohol-induced hepatitis
3. Drug-induced hepatitis
4. Bile duct obstruction
5. Autoimmune hepatitis
6. Disorders of bilirubin metabolism, such as Gilbert's syndrome

Investigations

1. CBC with DC
2. Total serum bilirubin, direct, and indirect
3. AST, ALT, GGT, alkaline phosphatase levels
4. USG of abdomen
5. Urinalysis
6. Prothrombin time, partial thromboplastin time
7. Viral hepatitis antigen assay for hepatitis A, B, C, D, E

Red Flags

1. A history of other autoimmune diseases, such as systemic lupus erythematosus or sclero-derma, is a red flag for hepatitis.
2. The use of acetaminophen, heavy metals, vitamin A, valproic acid, isoniazid, halothane, pyraz-inamide, rifampicin, over-the-counter natural or herbal preparations, troglitazone, or anabolic steroids can cause hepatitis.
3. People with a history of travel, unprotected sexual intercourse, or intravenous drug use and people in high-risk demographic groups such as health care workers are at risk for contract-ing hepatitis B.

Focused History

- Ask about the onset and duration of yellowness of the eyes, the color of stools and urine, any itching, fever, abdominal pain, bleeding tendencies, travel history, blood transfusion, detailed sexual history, medications, and social history.

Targeted Physical Examination

- General exam: look for yellowness of the sclera and palms as well as sores and general skin surface
- Abdominal exam: complete
- Brief CVS and RS exams

Case 19 Meddie Eurphy is a 55-year-old man with constipation.

Differential Diagnoses

1. Carcinoma of the colon
2. Hypothyroidism
3. Functional constipation
4. Drug-induced constipation
5. Depression
6. Diabetes mellitus
7. Anal fissure
8. Multiple sclerosis
9. Botulism
10. Chagas' disease
11. Intestinal obstruction

Investigations

1. Rectal exam
2. Fecal occult blood test
3. Anoscopy, proctoscopy
4. Stool culture with sensitivity testing
5. Abdominal x-ray
6. CBC with DC
7. Electrolytes
8. T_3, T_4, TSH levels
9. Colorectal transit study
10. Sigmoidoscopy
11. Colonoscopy

Red Flags

1. A history of a low-fiber diet may indicate functional constipation.

Focused History

- Inquire about the patient's normal bowel habits and any recent change.
- Inquire about the onset, frequency, and amount of stool passed, passed gas (for complete constipation or obstipation), tenesmus, episodes of diarrhea between bouts of constipation, vomiting, abdominal pain, and fever.
- Also ask about previous symptoms of depression and previous history of thyroid problems.

Targeted Physical Examination

- General exam, thyroid exam if history points to any thyroid disease
- Abdominal exam
- Brief CVS and RS exams

Case 20   Cameron Tiaz is a 20-year-old woman with complaints of lower abdominal pain, fever, and cervical discharge for 1 week.

Differential Diagnoses

1. Ectopic pregnancy
2. Intrauterine pregnancy
3. Pelvic inflammatory disease
4. Appendicitis
5. Ovarian cyst
6. Endometriosis
7. Salpingitis
8. Urinary tract infection

Investigations

1. Urine pregnancy test
2. CBC with DC
3. Electrolytes
4. Urinalysis
5. Urine culture with sensitivities
6. *Chlamydia,* gonorrhea test of cervical swab
7. RPR, VDRL tests for syphilis
8. Laparoscopy

Case 21   Brandy Arcia is a 60-year-old man with a history of peripheral vascular disease. He complains of an ulcer on his left leg with a purulent discharge.

Differential Diagnoses

1. Osteomyelitis
2. Aseptic ulceration
3. Cellulitis
4. Skin abscess
5. Venous ulcer
6. Arterial ulcer

Investigations

1. CBC with DC
2. Blood culture
3. ESR
4. CRP
5. X-ray of left lower limb
6. MRI
7. Bone scan
8. Biopsy of bone

Case 22   Halma Sayek is a 30-year-old woman with loose stools.

Differential Diagnoses

1. Viral diarrhea (rotavirus, Norwalk virus)
2. Bacterial diarrhea (*Campylobacter, Salmonella, Escherichia coli*)
3. Parasites (giardiasis, amebiasis)
4. Malabsorption (lactose intolerance, celiac sprue)
5. Inflammatory bowel disease
6. Drug-induced
7. Zollinger-Ellison syndrome
8. Laxative abuse
9. Chronic diarrhea (HIV)
10. Irritable bowel syndrome

Investigations

1. CBC with DC
2. Urinalysis
3. Stool for WBCs, culture with sensitivities, fat stain
4. Stool for ova and parasites
5. BUN, creatinine levels
6. Sigmoidoscopy
7. Colonoscopy

Red Flags

1. You must counsel patients with diarrhea about the importance of oral rehydration therapy. Some patients do not understand that they are supposed to drink plenty of fluids to prevent dehydration when they have diarrhea.

Focused History

■ Inquire about the onset, frequency, and amount of stool, whether stool floats in water, consistency, pain, bloody or mucoid stool, vomiting, fever, rashes, travel history, appetite and weight changes, and sexual history.

Targeted Physical Examination

■ General exam
■ Abdominal exam
■ CVS auscultation, RS auscultation (lung sounds)

Case 23   Kanna Oournikova is a 54-year-old woman who has not seen a doctor for the past 20 years. She is concerned about wrinkles in her face and wants your advice on Botox injections.

Differential Diagnoses

1. Normal routine exam
2. Breast carcinoma
3. Cervical carcinoma

DR|

4. Colon carcinoma
5. Hypertension
6. Diabetes mellitus
7. Hyperlipidemia
8. Anemia

Investigations

1. Breast exam
2. Pelvic exam
3. Pap smear
4. Mammogram
5. CBC with DC
6. Urinalysis
7. BUN, creatinine levels
8. Fasting blood sugar
9. Fasting lipid profile
10. Sigmoidoscopy, colonoscopy

Focused History

- After a detailed PMH you have to focus on areas specific for age and gender, and counsel the SP.

Targeted Physical Examination

- General exam
- Brief CVS, RS, and abdominal exams

Case 24   Armen Selectra is a 27-year-old woman with fever, headache, nausea, and photophobia, along with a history of sinusitis.

Differential Diagnoses

1. Meningitis (bacterial, viral, fungal)
2. Encephalitis
3. Brain abscess
4. Subarachnoid hemorrhage
5. CNS malignancy
6. Cerebral vasculitis
7. Endocarditis with emboli to CNS

Investigations

1. Lumbar puncture: cell count, Gram stain
2. Cerebrospinal fluid culture
3. Blood cultures
4. Head CT
5. CBC with DC
6. Chest x-ray
7. Urinalysis

8. Electrolytes
9. ESR

Red Flags

1. Recent otitis media, sinusitis, sick contacts, travel history, and an immunocompromised state are red flags.
2. Check for papilledema or focal neurologic deficit before doing a lumbar puncture.

Focused History

- Fever, nausea, neck stiffness, exposure to glaring lights, altered mental status, seizures

Targeted Physical Examination

- General exam
- CNS exam
- Ophthalmoscopic exam (for papilledema)
- Attempts to elicit Kernig's sign and Brudzinski's sign

Case 25 Gichard Rere is a 53-year-old man with fatigue, recurrent nose bleeds, and tachypnea who claims that he stopped picking his nose 20 years ago.

Differential Diagnoses

1. Occult malignancy
2. Leukemia
3. Leukemoid reaction
4. Infectious mononucleosis
5. Anemia
6. Diabetes mellitus

Investigations

1. CBC with DC
2. Electrolytes
3. Fecal occult blood test
4. Prothrombin time, partial thromboplastin time
5. Bleeding time, clotting time
6. Bone marrow biopsy
7. Chest x-ray
8. ECG
9. Absolute neutrophil count
10. Fasting blood sugar

Red Flags

1. Anemia, thrombocytopenia, and elevated WBCs with increased PT/PTT can occur in any of the above. A bone marrow biopsy is necessary for the diagnosis.
2. Cytogenetic studies and immunohistochemical testing are specific for acute myelogenous leukemia and acute lymphocytic leukemia.

Case 26 Jashley Hudd is a 24-year-old woman with headache, pain in the malar area, and a tenacious green mucoid discharge. She reports that over-the-counter decongestants are ineffective.

Differential Diagnoses

1. Sinusitis
2. Vasomotor rhinitis
3. Allergic rhinitis
4. Nasal polyps
5. Tumor
6. Cysts
7. Foreign body
8. Wegener's granulomatosis

Investigations

1. CBC with DC
2. Occipitomental x-ray (Waters' view)
3. Sinus aspiration and culture
4. CT scan
5. MRI
6. US
7. Diagnostic nasal endoscopy

Red Flags

1. Deviated nasal septum, dental abscess, trauma, foreign body, allergic rhinitis, and rapid changes in altitude predispose to acute sinusitis.
2. Sinusitis is a clinical diagnosis; investigations such as MRI and CT can be written to fill space.

Focused History

- History of pain, information about the nasal discharge, postnasal drip, any disorder of smell, fever, halitosis, watery eyes, epistaxis

Targeted Physical Examination

- General exam
- Examination of sinuses for tenderness
- Transillumination test
- Examination of oral cavity and throat for postnasal drip
- Brief CVS and RS exams

Case 27 Lennifer Hove Jewit is a 30-year-old woman with diarrhea.

Differential Diagnoses

1. Viral diarrhea (rotavirus, Norwalk virus)
2. Bacterial diarrhea (*Campylobacter, Shigella, Salmonella*)
3. Parasitic diarrhea (*Giardia*, amebiasis)
4. Malabsorption (lactose intolerance, celiac sprue)

5. Irritable bowel disease (Crohn's disease, ulcerative colitis)
6. Drug-induced diarrhea
7. Zollinger-Ellison syndrome
8. Laxative abuse
9. Chronic diarrhea (HIV)
10. Irritable bowel syndrome

Investigations

1. CBC with DC, electrolytes
2. Stool sample for WBCs, culture with sensitivity testing, fat stain
3. Stool sample for ova and parasites
4. Urinalysis
5. BUN, creatinine levels
6. Sigmoidoscopy, colonoscopy

Focused History

- Onset, frequency, and amount of stool, whether stool floats in water, consistency, pain, bloody or mucoid in nature, vomiting, fever, rashes, travel history, appetite and weight changes, sexual history

Targeted Physical Examination

- General exam
- Abdominal exam
- CVS auscultation, RS auscultation (lung sounds)

Case 28   Meve Startin is a 60-year-old man complaining of memory loss and progressive mental deterioration.

Differential Diagnoses

1. Alzheimer's dementia
2. Vitamin B_{12} deficiency
3. Brain tumor
4. Multi-infarct dementia
5. Subdural hematoma
6. Normal-pressure hydrocephalus
7. Electrolyte imbalance
8. Neurosyphilis
9. Creutzfeldt-Jakob disease

Investigations

1. CBC with DC, electrolytes
2. Urinalysis
3. Vitamin B_{12} levels
4. CT scan
5. EEG
6. VDRL test for syphilis

7. Lumbar puncture
8. Brain biopsy

Focused History

- Can the person remember recent events (is short-term memory impaired)? Or can the person remember events from further in the past (is long-term memory impaired)?
- Has the memory loss been getting worse over years?
- Has the memory loss been developing over weeks or months?
- Is the memory loss present all the time, or are there distinct episodes of amnesia? If there are amnesia episodes, how long do they last?
- Has there been a head injury in the recent past?
- Has the person experienced an event that was emotionally traumatic?
- Has the person undergone surgery or any procedure requiring a general anesthetic?
- Does the person use alcohol? How much?
- Does the person use illicit drugs? How much? What type?
- Is the person confused or disoriented?
- Can the person independently eat, dress, and perform similar self-care activities?
- Has the person had seizures?
- Use the mnemonic "SHEATH DRAFT".

Targeted Physical Examination

- General exam
- Detailed neurologic examination

Case 29 Ellen Unt is a 28-year-old woman with pain and tingling in the hand.

Differential Diagnoses

1. Carpal tunnel syndrome
2. Ulnar nerve injury
3. Fracture of scaphoid/colles
4. Gout/pseudogout/rheumatoid arthritis
5. Cervical radiculopathy
6. Raynaud's phenomenon
7. DeQuervain tenosynovitis

Investigations

1. CBC with DC
2. Electrolytes
3. X-ray of wrist
4. X-ray with carpal tunnel view
5. EMG
6. Bone scan
7. Nerve conduction study

Red Flags

1. Carpal tunnel syndrome most likely is due to a congenital predisposition. Other contributing factors include trauma or injury to the wrist that causes swelling, such as a sprain or a frac-

ture; overactivity of the pituitary gland; hypothyroidism; rheumatoid arthritis; mechanical problems in the wrist joint; work stress; repeated use of vibrating hand tools; fluid retention during pregnancy or menopause; or development of a cyst or tumor in the canal.

2. Women are three times more likely than men to develop carpal tunnel syndrome.

3. It is especially common in people performing assembly-line work such as manufacturing, sewing, finishing, cleaning, and meat, poultry, or fish packing. In fact, carpal tunnel syndrome is three times more common among assemblers than among data-entry personnel. A 2001 study that found heavy computer use (up to 7 hours per day) did not increase the risk of developing carpal tunnel syndrome.

Focused History

- Onset, limitation of activity, progression
- Occupational history (e.g., typing), trauma, rheumatoid arthritis, gout, renal disease, pregnancy, endocrine diseases
- Pain history

Targeted Physical Examination

- General exam
- Examine the hands, arms, shoulders, and neck.
- Examine the wrist for tenderness, swelling, warmth, and discoloration.
- Each finger should be tested for sensation, and the muscles at the base of the hand should be examined for strength and signs of atrophy.
- Tinel test: Tap on or press the median nerve area in the patient's wrist. The test is positive when tingling in the fingers or a resultant shocklike sensation occurs.
- Phalen, or wrist-flexion, test: Have the patient hold his or her forearms upright by pointing the fingers down and pressing the backs of the hands together. The presence of carpal tunnel syndrome is suggested if one or more symptoms, such as tingling or increasing numbness, are felt in the fingers within 1 minute.

Case 30 Hustin Doffman is a 70-year-old man complaining of frequent falls.

Differential Diagnoses

1. Dementia (Alzheimer's disease/multi-infarct dementia)
2. Transient ischemic attack
3. Cerebellar disease
4. Depression
5. Parkinson's disease
6. Cataract
7. Hypoglycemia
8. Orthostatic hypotension
9. Heart block
10. Stroke
11. Drug-induced dementia

Investigations

1. CBC with DC
2. Electrolytes
3. Urinalysis
4. Blood sugar level
5. ECG
6. Tilt table study
7. CT scan
8. MRI

Case 31   Memi Doore is a 40-year-old woman who complains of lack of energy and difficulty sleeping.

Differential Diagnoses

1. Endogenous depression
2. Grieving/bereavement
3. Bipolar disorder
4. Drug-induced lethargy
5. Substance abuse
6. Hypothyroidism
7. Postpartum depression

Investigations

1. CBC with DC
2. Electrolytes
3. TSH, T_3, T_4 levels
4. CT scan
5. MRI
6. Dexamethasone suppression test
7. MHPG levels
8. AST, ALT levels

Focused History

- Is the problem loss of energy or boredom?
- Is there unusual fatigability?
- How has the sleep pattern changed recently?
- What exactly is the sleep problem? (Difficulty in falling sleep or early awakening?)
- Is drowsiness present during the day?
- Obtain history of medication use, including sleeping pills.
- Use the mnemonic "SIGE CAPS".

Targeted Physical Examination

- General exam
- Brief CVS, RS, and thyroid exams

Case 32 Mrs. Smith complains that her 8-month-old child has fever, rash, and convulsions.

Differential Diagnoses

1. Viral exanthems (measles, mumps, rubella, chickenpox)
2. Meningitis
3. Febrile seizures
4. Otitis media
5. Urinary tract infection
6. Streptococcal sore throat
7. Kawasaki's syndrome
8. Tonsillitis/pharyngitis

Investigations

1. CBC with DC
2. Electrolytes
3. Urinalysis and urine culture with sensitivities
4. Lumbar puncture
5. Sputum culture with sensitivity testing
6. Chest x-ray
7. Monospot test
8. Rapid streptococcal test
9. Blood cultures

Focused History

- Onset of fever and its progression, response to medications
- Seizures: onset, spreading, bowel/bladder incontinence, postictal state
- Cough, ear discharge, diarrhea, vomiting
- Rash: onset, location, extent and spread, itching and pain over rash
- ABCDEFGHIJK mnemonic for pediatric history

Targeted Physical Examination

- Request physical exam of the baby.
- In this case, counseling the mother/caregiver becomes very important.

Case 33 Rulia Joberts is a 40-year-old woman with weight loss for the past 3 months.

Differential Diagnoses

1. Depression
2. Diabetes
3. Hyperthyroidism
4. Anorexia nervosa/bulimia
5. Occult malignancy
6. Substance abuse
7. Drug-induced weight loss
8. Malnutrition
9. Infectious disease (tuberculosis, HIV)

Investigations

1. CBC with DC
2. Electrolytes
3. TSH, T$_3$, T$_4$ levels
4. Enzyme-linked immunosorbent assay (ELISA)
5. Endoscopy
6. Colonoscopy
7. Fecal occult blood test
8. ESR
9. C-reactive protein

Red Flags

1. Deliberate self-starvation with weight loss, fear of gaining weight, refusal to eat, denial of hunger, constant exercising, greater amounts of hair on the body or the face, sensitivity to cold temperatures, absent or irregular periods, loss of scalp hair, and self-perception of being fat when the person is really too thin indicate anorexia nervosa
2. Eating disorders usually arise in adolescence and disproportionately affect females. Death may occur from starvation, suicide, or electrolyte imbalance.

Case 34   Candy Awford is a 30-year-old woman complaining of weight gain.

Differential Diagnoses

1. Excess food intake
2. Sedentary lifestyle
3. Polycystic ovarian disease
4. Hypothyroidism
5. Depression
6. Cushing's syndrome
7. Drug-induced weight gain (corticosteroids, lithium, tricyclic antidepressant)

Investigations

1. CBC with DC
2. Electrolytes
3. Dexamethasone suppression test, 24-hour urine cortisol
4. TSH, T$_3$, T$_4$ levels
5. Lipid profile
6. Liver function tests
7. Blood sugar
8. Skin-fold thickness

Encounter Counseling

The patient may ask, "*Why lose weight?*"

You can answer like this: "*Being overweight increases the risk of developing a number of serious medical conditions, such as coronary heart disease, type 2 diabetes, high cholesterol, high blood pressure, breathing disorders during sleep, some types of cancer, osteoarthritis, gallstones, certain forms of urinary incontinence, and menstrual irregularities. In addition, for people who already have coronary heart disease, type 2 diabetes, high cholesterol, or high blood pressure, being overweight increases the dangers of the underlying condition. Fortunately, if you are concerned about these health risks, there are a number of specific steps you can take to improve your health."*

Also, advise the SP about eating better and changing dietary habits. You may refer the SP to a nutrition specialist, such as a registered dietitian, for in-depth counseling about food choices. You may also offer some simple practical advice, such as *"Don't use a remote control when watching TV. Simply getting up to change the channel can make a difference in your activity level."* Also, you can inform the SP about weight-loss programs and weight-loss medications.

Case 35   Brock Hudson is a 36-year-old man who was diagnosed with HIV 3 years ago. He comes to your office for a drug refill.

Differential Diagnoses

You are looking for the complications of HIV.

1. Candidiasis
2. Tuberculosis
3. Herpes simplex/zoster
4. Hairy leukoplakia
5. Kaposi's sarcoma
6. Pneumocystis carinii/jiroveci pneumonia
7. Toxoplasmosis
8. Coccidioidomycosis
9. Cryptosporidiosis
10. Disseminated *Mycobacterium avium* complex
11. Histoplasmosis
12. Cytomegalovirus retinitis
13. CNS lymphoma

Investigations

1. CBC with DC
2. CD4 count
3. HIV RNA viral load
4. Chest x-ray
5. Purified protein derivative test
6. RPR/VDRL tests for syphilis
7. IgG serology (*Toxoplasma* and cytomegalovirus)
8. Hepatitis B surface antigen
9. Anal swabs

Red Flags

1. Counseling the patient is the most important aspect in a case like this one. You must indicate the importance of safe sexual practices, medication compliance/adherence, proper vaccination, and avoidance of intravenous drug use.
2. Inform the patient about HIV support groups, and advise the patient not to donate blood or organs.

Focused History

- Ask about medications currently taken, compliance, and adverse effects of the drugs.
- Ask about shortness of breath, fever, headache, eye problems, gastritis, oral ulcers, dysphagia, odynophagia, skin rash, diarrhea, urethral discharge.
- Ask also about symptoms of depression.
- Obtain a detailed sexual history.
- Specifically ask if he has informed all his partners about his HIV status.
- Counsel about safe sexual practices and the availability of support groups.

Targeted Physical Examination

- General exam
- Eye examination with ophthalmoscope
- Oral cavity exam, cervical lymph nodes exam
- Brief CVS, RS, and abdominal exams

Case 36   Amela Panderson is a 52-year-old woman complaining of dyspareunia.

Differential Diagnoses

1. Menopause
2. Trauma
3. Vaginisimus
4. Vulvodynia
5. Endometriosis
6. Retroverted uterus
7. Iatrogenic (pelvic surgery)

Investigations

1. Pelvic exam
2. CBC with DC
3. Electrolytes
4. Urinalysis
5. Follicle-stimulating hormone, luteinizing hormone
6. Vaginal/cervical cultures
7. PAP smear

Red Flags

1. Menopause; obstetric delivery; a history of lacerations, episiotomies, or other trauma; a history of STDs or sexual or physical abuse; depression; or anxiety disorders can cause dyspareunia.

Focused History

- Pain history: When is the onset of the pain—before, during, or after entry, with deep penetration? Is the pain vaginal?
- Is the pain pruritic, burning, or aching in quality?
- Are there other sexual dysfunctions, such as arousal, lubrication, or orgasmic difficulties?

- Does the patient experience bowel or bladder symptoms?
- Are there vaginal symptoms, including discharge, burning, or itching?
- Does the patient have a history of STDs, especially with herpes simplex virus or human papillomavirus?
- Is there an obstetric delivery history of lacerations, episiotomies, or other trauma?
- Is there a history of abdominal or genitourinary surgery or radiation?
- Has the patient had prior gynecologic diagnoses, including endometriosis, fibroids, or chronic pelvic pain?
- What is the patient's current contraception method? Is there any history of intrauterine device use?
- What is the patient's view of the problem?
- Has the problem been present in other relationships?
- Are the partners able to discuss the problem? If so, what actions have they tried?
- Is there any history of sexual or physical abuse?
- To what extent are other life stressors a factor?
- Is there evidence of depression or anxiety disorders?

Targeted Physical Examination

- General exam
- Abdominal exam
- Brief neuropsychiatric exam

Case 37   Tuma Hurman is the mother of a 1-week-old boy who is yellow in color.

Differential Diagnoses

1. Physiologic jaundice
2. Breast milk jaundice
3. Hemoglobinopathies
4. Neonatal infection
5. Biliary tract obstruction
6. Kernicterus
7. Hypercarotinemia

Investigations

1. Examination of the child
2. CBC with DC
3. Electrolytes
4. Urinalysis
5. Bilirubin levels (direct, indirect, total)
6. Coombs test
7. Hemoglobin electrophoresis
8. Liver function tests
9. US of abdomen
10. HIDA scan

Red Flags

1. Jaundice on the first day of life is not physiologic. "Physiologic" jaundice occurs after the first day of life and within 1 week after birth.
2. Kernicterus results from irreversible deposition of bilirubin in the basal ganglia and is potentially fatal.

Focused History

- ABCDEFGHIJK mnemonic for pediatric history, used appropriately
- Fever, congenital malformation, breast-feeding, birth trauma, enlargement of abdomen, history of lethargy, high-pitched cry, seizures, and so on
- Any vaccination, medications given

Targeted Physical Examination

- General exam

Case 38   Gel Mibson complains that his 9-year-old daughter is shorter than her peers.

Differential Diagnoses

1. Constitutional delay
2. Familial short stature
3. Hypothyroidism
4. Deprivation dwarfism
5. Chronic disease (brain tumor, bowel disease, type 1 diabetes, renal tubular acidosis, rickets)
6. Turner's syndrome

Investigations

1. Examination of the child
2. CBC with DC
3. Electrolytes with calcium and phosphate
4. ESR
5. TSH, T_3, T_4 levels
6. U/A
7. X-rays of hand and wrist
8. Insulin growth factor-1 levels over 24 hours

Red Flags

1. It is possible that the SP may bring a growth chart for you to interpret. If not, you must ask the SP to bring it.

Case 39   Tohn Javoltra is a 40-year-old man complaining of fatigue.

Differential Diagnoses

1. Depression
2. Anemia
3. Cancer
4. Chemotherapy
5. Infectious diseases (HIV, EBV)
6. Hyperglycemia
7. Chronic fatigue syndrome
8. Multiple sclerosis
9. Parkinson's disease

Investigations

1. CBC with DC
2. Electrolytes
3. Blood sugar
4. ELISA
5. CT
6. MRI
7. Urinalysis
8. Monospot test

Red Flags

1. Tiredness with lack of energy is a *universal* complaint.

Focused History

- History of fatigue, sleep pattern changes, medications, treatment for any disease, onset, suicidal ideation
- Use SIGE CAPS mnemonic.

Targeted Physical Examination

- General exam
- Brief CVS, RS, and CNS exams

Case 40   George Gloomy is a 42-year-old man complaining of excessive daytime sleepiness and insomnia.

Differential Diagnoses

1. Inadequate sleep
2. Poor sleep quality
3. Drug-induced sleepiness/insomnia
4. Narcolepsy
5. Restless leg syndrome

6. Environmental influences
7. Hyperthyroidism

Investigations

1. CBC with DC
2. ECG
3. Electrolytes
4. Blood glucose
5. Sleep study
6. TSH, T_3, T_4 levels
7. Urinalysis
8. Urine toxicology screen

Red Flags

1. Obesity, male gender, oropharyngeal abnormalities, smoking, snoring, restlessness, nocturia, and gastroesophageal reflux disease can cause difficulty in sleeping at night and must be asked about in the history.
2. Pain that is worse with immobility and relieved with activity indicates restless leg syndrome, also known as periodic limb movement disorder. This disorder is associated with caffeine intake, iron deficiency, renal failure, fibromyalgia, and pregnancy.
3. Drugs such as antidepressants, steroids, caffeine, alcohol, stimulants, decongestants, steroids, and bronchodilators can cause insomnia.
4. Poor sleep quality can be due to obstructive or central sleep apnea.
5. Stress, working the graveyard shift, and social factors can cause inadequate sleep.

Case 41   Jeeter Pennings is a 52-year-old man who comes to your clinic for his health checkup. He has a history of hypertension for the past 15 years and currently takes atenolol and captopril. He indicates that he wants to stop taking his antihypertensive medications because his blood pressure is "good."

Differential Diagnoses

You are looking for the complications of hypertension:
1. Hypertensive retinopathy
2. Hypertensive nephropathy
3. Hypertensive encephalopathy
4. Transient ischemic attack/cerebrovascular accident
5. Peripheral vascular disease
6. Coronary artery disease
7. Accelerated hypertension
8. Arrhythmia
9. Congestive cardiac failure

Investigations

1. CBC with DC
2. BUN, creatinine levels
3. Electrolytes

4. Urinalysis
5. ECG
6. Fasting blood sugar
7. Lipid profile

 ### Red Flags

1. Any personal history of cardiac disease, diabetes mellitus, stroke, elevated cholesterol, gout, recent weight changes, and renal disease must be discussed.
2. Ask about prior medications, side effects, and response.
3. Advise about dietary, exercise, and social habits.
4. Advise about over-the-counter medications that may exacerbrate hypertension, such as OCPs, NSAIDs, steroids, and decongestants.
5. A funduscopic exam is a must. Listen for abdominal bruit for renal artery stenosis. The cardiac examination must be complete.

Focused History

- Age at onset
- Associated symptoms such as headache, dizziness, blurring vision, chest pain, palpitations
- Regular blood pressure checkups, medication compliance
- Ask if urinalysis, blood sugar, and cholesterol level tests have been done.

Targeted Physical Examination

- Note the recorded blood pressure from the doorway information, and inform patient about the reading. If instructed, record the blood pressure in different postures: lying, sitting.
- General exam
- Ophthalmoscopic exam
- Brief CVS, RS, and abdominal exams
- Check pulses

Case 42   Roxanne Starr is a 40-year-old obese woman with right upper quadrant pain, fever, and emesis.

Differential Diagnoses

1. Acute cholecystitis
2. Cholelithiasis
3. Cholangitis
4. Pancreatitis
5. Peptic ulcer disease
6. Renal colic
7. Viral hepatitis
8. Ruptured ovarian cyst
9. Ectopic pregnancy

Investigations

1. Rectal/pelvic exam
2. CBC with DC

3. Electrolytes
4. Urinalysis
5. X-ray of abdomen (erect), chest x-ray (erect)
6. US of abdomen
7. ERCP
8. Amylase, lipase levels
9. AST, ALT, alkaline phosphatase, GGT, bilirubin levels
10. HIDA scan
11. Pregnancy test
12. Hepatitis panel

Red Flags

1. The 6 Fs—fat, female, forty, flatulent, fertile, now with fever—point to the diagnosis of acute cholecystitis.
2. Fever, right upper quadrant pain, and jaundice combine to form Charcot's triad for ascending cholangitis. With the addition of mental status changes and hypotension, the triad becomes Reynauld's pentad.
3. Murphy's sign should be elicited.

Focused History

- LIQOR DRAW mnemonic for pain history.
- Ask about vomiting, fever, last menstrual period, vaginal discharge, vaginal bleeding.

Targeted Physical Examination

- General exam
- Abdominal exam (important to check for costovertebral angle tenderness)
- Attempts to elicit Murphy's sign
- Quick auscultation of heart and lung sounds

Case 43   Fristina Cingulara is a 28-year-old woman with pain in her right flank.

Differential Diagnoses

1. Renal calculi
2. Trauma
3. Obstructive uropathy
4. Pancreatitis
5. Perinephric abcess
6. Polycystic kidney disease
7. Pyelonephritis
8. Renal cell carcinoma
9. Renal infarction
10. Renal vein thrombosis
11. Ectopic pregnancy
12. Twisted ovarian cyst

Investigations

1. CBC with DC
2. Electrolytes
3. US of abdomen
4. CT/MRI of abdomen
5. Input/output charting
6. X-ray of abdomen
7. Intravenous pyelography
8. Cystoscopy
9. Voiding cystourethrography
10. Pregnancy test

Red Flags

1. Pain starting from the loin to the groin, with nausea and vomiting, is suggestive of renal calculi. Check for costovertebral angle tenderness.
2. Weight loss with hematuria suggests renal cell carcinoma.
3. Positive family history for polycystic kidney disease.

Focused History

- Use LIQOR DRAW mnemonic for pain history.
- Does the patient's face ever look puffy in the morning? Are the ankles swollen?
- Urinary symptoms with complete history:

  - ☐ Is the urine altered in amount or color?
  - ☐ Is the urine frothy, or is there any blood in it?
  - ☐ Is there any pain during micturition?
  - ☐ If so, does the pain occur before, during, or after the act?

Targeted Physical Examination

- General exam: look for puffiness of face, pallor, and ankle edema
- Abdominal exam with check for costovertebral angle tenderness
- Brief CVS and RS exams

Case 44   Aniffer Janiston is a 22-year-old woman who presents in the ED with right lower abdominal pain and lack of appetite.

Differential Diagnoses

1. Acute appendicitis
2. Ruptured ectopic pregnancy
3. Pelvic inflammatory disease
4. Urinary tract infection
5. Twisted ovarian cyst
6. Urethral stone
7. Acute lymphatic mesenteritis
8. Acute gastroenteritis

Investigations

1. CBC with DC
2. Rectal exam
3. Pelvic exam
4. Urinalysis
5. X-ray of abdomen
6. US of abdomen
7. Barium enema
8. CT scan of abdomen
9. Pregnancy test

Red Flags

1. Right lower quadrant pain aggravated by motion or cough, anorexia, nausea, vomiting, urinary frequency, and dysuria point to acute appendicitis. The diagnosis is primarily based on physical examination. Murphy's sign must be elicited to make the diagnosis. The psoas sign and obturator sign should also be elicited.

Focused History

- LIQOR DRAW mnemonic for pain history.
- Ask about vomiting, fever, last menstrual period, vaginal discharge, vaginal bleeding.

Targeted Physical Examination

- General exam
- Abdominal exam with check for costovertebral angle tenderness
- Tests for psoas sign and obturator sign
- Brief CVS and RS exams

Case 45 Evita Scleron is a 44-year-old woman complaining that she was a victim of domestic abuse.

Differential Diagnoses

1. Domestic violence
2. Posttraumatic stress disorder (PTSD)
3. Sexual assault
4. Somatoform disorder
5. Dissociative disorder
6. Malingering

Investigations

1. Pelvic exam
2. Rectal exam
3. CBC with DC
4. Pap smear
5. Electrolytes
6. Relevant radiographs
7. Prothrombin time, partial thromboplastin time

Red Flags

1. Use the mnemonic SAVED in your history.
2. The SP may present with different patterns of bruises that were artificially reproduced. You must document these bruises and ask permission to photograph them.
3. Neuropsychiatric assessment is a must.
4. Counseling should be done with regard to support systems available and emergency plan.
5. If patient is older than 60 years or younger than 18 years, it is imperative that you include in your patient note that you will contact the appropriate authorities.

Focused History

- SAVED mnemonic.
- Ask about partner's alcohol use/drug history.
- Ask if there are any weapons at home.
- Ask about other social problems.
- Obtain the sexual history.

Targeted Physical Examination

- General exam
- Examination for bruises or fractures of limbs
- Brief CVS and CNS exams

Case 46   Billy Bob Borton is a 47-year-old man complaining of bad breath.

Differential Diagnoses

1. Common cold
2. Gastric carcinoma
3. Esophageal carcinoma
4. Hepatic encephalopathy
5. Ketoacidosis
6. Bowel obstruction
7. Lung abscess
8. Periodontal disease
9. Ozena
10. Pharyngitis
11. Zenker's diverticulum

Investigations

1. Rectal exam
2. CBC with DC
3. Electrolytes
4. Chest x-ray
5. Barium swallow exam
6. EGD
7. Blood glucose

Red Flags

1. History of undigested regurgitated food indicates Zenker's diverticulum.
2. A history of weight loss, dysphagia, and achalasia may indicate carcinoma.
3. Poor dental hygiene predisposes to periodontal diseases.
4. More than 90 million people suffer from chronic halitosis or bad breath. In most cases it originates from the gums and tongue. The odor is caused by bacteria from the decay of food particles, other debris in the mouth, and poor oral hygiene.
5. Bad breath is primarily caused by poor oral hygiene, medical infection, gum disease, diabetes, kidney failure, or liver malfunction. Xerostoma (dry mouth) and tobacco use also contribute to this problem. Cancer patients who undergo radiation therapy may experience dry mouth.
6. Even stress, dieting, snoring, age, and hormonal changes can have an effect on the breath
7. Counsel patient to brush twice a day with fluoride toothpaste to remove food debris and plaque. Patient should brush the tongue, and once a day should use floss or an interdental cleaner to clean between teeth.

Case 47   James Dameron is a 27-year-old man complaining of hiccups (also known as singultus).

Differential Diagnoses

1. Abdominal distention
2. Gastritis
3. Gastric dilation
4. Increased intracranial pressure
5. Brainstem lesion
6. Pancreatitis
7. Pleural irritation
8. Renal failure
9. Abdominal surgery

Investigations

1. CBC with DC
2. Electrolytes
3. X-ray of the abdomen
4. EGD
5. CT of the abdomen
6. CT of the head
7. Amylase, lipase levels
8. BUN, creatinine levels

Red Flags

1. Singultus can result from any of the above conditions. Anything that causes irritation to the esophagus can cause it.
2. Counsel the patient about dietary modifications.
3. The exact cause remains a mystery despite centuries of contemplation. Medical training is not required to diagnose hiccups. Brief episodes that self-terminate or respond to simple maneuvers need no investigation or follow-up care.

4. In contrast, persistent and intractable hiccups frequently are associated with an underlying pathologic process and may induce significant morbidity. The focus of the history, examination, and investigation is to identify these causes and effects.
5. Hiccups that abate with sleep and are temporally related to stressful circumstances commonly are psychogenic in origin.
6. Arrhythmia-induced syncope has been reported as both a cause and an effect of hiccups.
7. Gastroesophageal reflux may cause or result from hiccups.
8. Weight loss, insomnia, and emotional distress may complicate prolonged episodes.
9. A full systemic inquiry, surgical history, and comprehensive drug history may reveal one of the many causes.
10. Alcoholism may contribute to the development of hiccups.

Targeted Physical Examination

- General exam
- Brief CVS, RS, and abdominal exams

Case 48   Celine De Old is a 34-year-old woman complaining of horseness of the voice.

Differential Diagnoses

1. Vocal cord polyp/nodule
2. Hypothyroidism
3. Gastroesophageal reflux disease
4. Laryngitis
5. Laryngeal leukoplakia
6. Sjögren's syndrome
7. Thoracic aortic aneurysm
8. Inhalation injury

Investigations

1. CBC with DC
2. Electrolytes
3. Indirect laryngoscopy
4. Fiberoptic laryngoscopy
5. TSH, T_3, T_4
6. Anti-Rho (sicca syndrome A), anti-La (sicca syndrome B)
7. Chest x-ray
8. CT scan chest

Red Flags

1. "Singer's," "screamer's," or "teacher's nodules" are mostly due to voice strain. A susceptible person may be a pop singer who with an untrained voice or poor technique uses falsetto voice on occasion.
2. Immediately advise the patient to cancel all performances.

Focused History

- Any pain in the throat, occupational history, misuse of voice, any other speech problems

Targeted Physical Examination

- General exam
- Brief CVS and RS exams
- Oral exam

Case 49 Dobert Role is a 48-year-old man complaining of impotence and wants you to prescribe Viagra.

Differential Diagnoses

1. Peripheral neuropathy
2. Psychological origin
3. Trauma
4. Leriche's syndrome
5. Alcohol
6. Smoking
7. Iatrogenic
8. CNS lesion
9. Peyronie's disease
10. Drug-induced impotence

Investigations

1. CBC with DC
2. Electrolytes
3. Pelvic exam
4. Postage-stamp test
5. CT of head
6. Blood glucose level
7. Urinalysis
8. Urine toxicology screen
9. Doppler study

Red Flags

1. You must first distinguish between primary and secondary impotence.
2. It is imperative that you ensure privacy, confirm confidentiality, and establish a rapport between yourself and the patient.
3. Ask about a history of diabetes mellitus, which can cause peripheral neuropathy.
4. Atenolol, amitriptyline, carbamazepine, digoxin, imipramine, prazosin, thiazide diuretics, cimetidine, escitalopram, and tranylcipramine are drugs known to cause impotence.

Focused History

- Onset of the impotence, problems with sexual disease/arousal or ejaculation, continuous or intermittent pain in legs and buttocks
- Anxiety, depression symptoms, thyroid disease, diabetes, hypertension, trauma, drugs
- Detailed sexual history, including number of partners, conflicts with partner

Targeted Physical Examination

- General exam
- Feel for pulses in both lower limbs.

Case 50 Hugh Brant is a 31-year-old man who has pain on the left side of his face.

Differential Diagnoses

1. Trigeminal neuralgia
2. Sphenopalatine neuralgia
3. Postherpetic neuralgia
4. Herpes zoster oticus
5. Glossopharyngeal neuralgia
6. Temporomandibular joint syndrome
7. Multiple sclerosis
8. Sinusitis
9. Dental caries
10. Acute glaucoma
11. Trauma

Investigations

1. CBC with DC
2. Electrolytes
3. X-ray (Waters' view)
4. CT of head
5. MRI of head
6. Tzanck test
7. Tonometry

Red Flags

1. Pain triggered by touching the nose and cheek area or on exposure to hot or cold environments indicates trigeminal neuralgia. Affected patients do not shave that area of the face.
2. Multiple neurologic deficits are present in multiple sclerosis.
3. Trismus, malocclusion, clicking, and crepitus are seen in temporomandibular joint syndrome.
4. Vesicles in the ear canal and oral mucosa with pain along a single dermatome indicate herpes reactivation.
5. In sinusitis, patients experience pain when they bend over.
6. Poor oral hygiene predisposes to dental caries.

Focused History

- LIQOR DRAW mnemonic for pain history
- Specific trigger factors (e.g., washing, chewing, brushing, laughing, swallowing, coughing)
- Any earache
- Any fever, headache, nausea, vomiting

Targeted Physical Examination

- General exam
- CNS exam: trigeminal nerve exam
- Oral exam
- Temporomandibular joint exam

Case 51   Tina Mourner is a 17-year-old girl who has never had a menstrual period.

Differential Diagnoses

1. Müllerian agenesis
2. Androgen insensitivity
3. Turner's syndrome
4. Imperforate hymen
5. Pregnancy
6. Gonadal dysgenesis
7. Hypothalamic-pituitary-ovarian (HPO) axis failure
8. Adrenal tumor
9. Hypothyroidism
10. Polycystic ovarian disease

Investigations

1. Breast exam
2. Pelvic exam
3. Serum testosterone levels
4. US of abdomen/pelvis
5. Karyotype
6. Follicle-stimulating hormone (FSH), luteinizing hormone levels
7. Beta-human chorionic gonadotropin level

Red Flags

1. Normal breast development + absence of uterus + presence of pubic/axillary hair = müllerian agenesis
2. Absence of pubic/axillary hair + increased testosterone + 46XY karyotype = androgen insensitivity
3. Absence of breasts + presence of uterus + increased FSH level + 46X karyotype = Turner's syndrome
4. Decreased FSH level + 46XX karyotype = HPO failure

Focused History

- Ask about previous cycle, if any.
- Ask about vaginal bleeding or any visual changes.
- Discuss the chance of getting pregnant.
- Obtain detailed obstetric/gynecologic and sexual histories.
- Ask whether there is any similar condition in the family history.

Targeted Physical Examination

- General exam
- Abdominal exam

Case 52   Becky Harpe is a 37-year-old woman complaining of postcoital bleeding.

Differential Diagnoses

1. Cervicitis
2. Human papillomavirus
3. Endometriosis
4. Cervical dysplasia
5. Herpes simplex virus
6. Trauma
7. Foreign body

Investigations

1. Pelvic exam
2. Pap smear
3. CBC with DC
4. Electrolytes
5. BUN, creatinine levels
6. Urinalysis
7. Cervical biopsy and culture

Red Flags

1. Postcoital bleeding in the perimenopausal age group is cervical carcinoma until proved otherwise. Therefore, metastatic workup must include cystoscopy, proctoscopy, intravenous pyelography, chest x-ray, and CT of abdomen/pelvis.
2. The most common cause of cervicitis is chlamydial or gonorrheal infection.
3. Counsel the patient about routine Pap smear, mammography, and safe sexual practices.
4. The risk of cervical dysplasia increases with multiple sexual partners, sex before age 18, childbirth before age 16, or a history of STDs.
5. Chlamydial infection, gonorrhea, and trichomoniasis are usually sexually transmitted diseases.
6. Uterine polyps occur when the endometrium overgrows, causing protrusions into the uterus. The patient experiences metorrhagia. Other symptoms include vaginal bleeding after sex, spotting, menorrhagia, bleeding after menopause, and breakthrough bleeding during hormone therapy.
7. Uterine fibroid tumors are solid masses made of fibrous tissue. In women who can wait until menopause, fibroids shrink and disappear once the body stops producing estrogen. It is important that women with fibroids never take estrogen in any form, including birth control pills, since estrogen increases fibroid growth.

Case 53   Bule Brenner is a 68-year-old man complaining of difficulty swallowing solids and a 15-pound weight loss. He has a 40-pack-year smoking history.

Differential Diagnoses

1. Esophageal carcinoma
2. Gastric carcinoma

3. Achalasia cardia
4. Scleroderma
5. Diffuse esophageal spasm
6. Esophageal diverticula
7. Peptic stricture
8. Esophageal web
9. Schatzki's ring
10. Esophagitis

Investigations

1. CBC with DC
2. Electrolytes, serum calcium level
3. Chest x-ray
4. Barium swallow
5. Upper endoscopy with biopsy
6. CT scan of chest
7. ECG
8. Endoscopic US

Red Flags

1. Dysphagia initially with liquids and later with solids + weight loss + anemia + recent onset of symptoms = esophageal carcinoma.
2. Iron deficiency anemia + esophageal web + spoon-shaped nails = Plummer-Vinson syndrome (a.k.a. Patterson-Kelly syndrome).
3. Dysphagia for liquids and solids with a longstanding history indicates achalasia.
4. Systemic manifestations and tightening of the skin in the setting of heartburn suggest scleroderma.

Focused History

- Is swallowing difficult or painful?
- Where does the food appear to stick?
- Is it worse with solids or liquids, and which came first?
- Is there any heartburn?
- Ask about chest pain.
- Ask about excessive secretion of saliva with regurgitation of fluids.
- Ask about appetite, vomiting, constipation, diarrhea, or enlargement of lymph nodes (use the term "swollen glands").
- Inquire into alcohol use and smoking history.

Targeted Physical Examination

- General exam: pallor + lymph nodes
- Brief CVS and RS exams
- Oral exam
- Abdominal exam

Case 54   Kevin Jostner is a 51-year-old man with an increased urge to void urine.

Differential Diagnoses

1. Benign prostatic hypertrophy
2. Bladder calculi
3. Bladder carcinoma
4. Prostatic carcinoma
5. Multiple sclerosis
6. Reiter's syndrome
7. Spinal cord compression
8. Urinary tract infection
9. Urethral stricture
10. Medication

Investigations

1. Rectal exam
2. Urinalysis, urine culture with sensitivity testing
3. CBC with DC
4. Electrolytes
5. BUN, creatinine levels
6. Intravenous pyelogram
7. US of abdomen/pelvis
8. Cystoscopy
9. Cystometry
10. Postvoid residual work-up

Red Flags

1. Increased urinary frequency, nocturia, incontinence, and hematuria suggest benign prostatic hypertrophy. Initially patients have symptoms of prostatism: decreased caliber and force of urine, urinary hesitancy, inability to start or stop the act of voiding, and urine retention.
2. Anxiety neurosis is suggested by headache, diaphoresis, hyperventilation, palpitation, muscle spasm, genitourinary and gastrointestinal complaints.

Focused History

- Is the patient able to void urine?
- Is the patient able to hold urine?
- Is the stream of urine normal or reduced in flow?
- Is the urine altered in color and amount?
- Is there increased volume? If so, is it increased by day or night?
- Is increased volume associated with thirst?
- Is there any pain during micturition?

Targeted Physical Examination

- General exam
- Abdominal exam with check for costovertebral angle tenderness
- Brief CVS and RS exams

Case 55   Jim Marry is a 46-year-old man complaining of unsteadiness and instability.

Differential Diagnoses

1. Stroke
2. Wernicke's encephalopathy
3. Spinocerebellar ataxia/cerebellar hemorrhage
4. Cranial trauma
5. Diabetic neuropathy
6. Encephalomyelitis
7. Guillain-Barré syndrome/multiple sclerosis/Friedreich's ataxia
8. Metastatic carcinoma/posterior fossa tumor
9. Syringomyelia
10. Drug-induced unsteadiness

Investigations

1. CBC with DC
2. Electrolytes
3. Blood sugar level
4. BUN, creatinine levels
5. CT scan of head
6. MRI of head
7. Urine/serum toxicology screen

Red Flags

1. Have the patient walk from one end of the room to the other. Ensure patient safety. Provide the option of a cane or walker.
2. Counsel patient about home care, and especially about potential hazards in the home.
3. Ataxia with or without unilateral or bilateral motor weakness + loss of consciousness = vestibular basilar insufficiency/stroke.
4. Gait abnormalities + truncal/limb ataxia worsening with time + vomiting/headache/papilledema/vertigo/occulomotor-sensory-motor deficits = posterior fossa tumor.

Focused History

- Is the problem loss of balance, vertigo, or dizziness?
- Was it sudden in onset?
- Was it associated with weakness, visual disturbance, or sensory loss on one side of the body?
- Was it associated with headache?
- Ask about history of heart disease or any other vascular disease.
- Ask about tremor, speech disturbance, impairment of memory.
- Ask about exposure to toxic substances.

Targeted Physical Examination

- General exam
- Complete CNS exam
- Auscultation of heartbeat

Case 56 Martha Beuhart is a 38-year-old woman who claims that she has been sexually assaulted.

Differential Diagnoses

1. Rape
2. Posttraumatic stress disorder
3. Dissociative disorder
4. Domestic violence
5. Malingering
6. Somatoform disorder

Investigations

1. Pelvic exam
2. Pap smear
3. Wood's light exam for semen
4. Saline sample from mouth, anus, and cervix
5. VDRL test for syphilis, HIV, hepatitis B screening
6. Beta-human chorionic gonadotropin level
7. Inform local authorities

Red Flags

1. Ask the patient's permission to perform an HIV test.
2. Obtain a reproductive, obstetric, sexual, and contraceptive history.
3. Stabilize the patient and counsel the patient about local support groups.
4. The victim may be overwhelmed by confusing emotions—fear, grief, guilt, shame, rage.
5. Support groups can help to the victim deal with feelings of isolation, secrecy, and shame.
6. Young people ages 12 to 24 years are the group most likely to be victims of crimes such as rape, assault, and robbery. Many of these crimes occur at school, on the street, or at a park or playground.
7. Sexual assault may include sexual touching, vaginal penetration, sexual intercourse, rape, and attempted rape.
8. Drugs sometimes used to assist a sexual assault are GHB (gamma-hydroxybutyric acid), flunitrazepam, and ketamine.

Focused History

- Is there any history of being unable to sleep at night and unable to stay awake during the day, or trouble thinking clearly, concentrating, and making decisions?
- Is the patient experiencing any fear, anxiety, or guilt?
- Were any drugs used to assist the sexual assault?
- Were there any physical, emotional, or sexual problems during this time, even if the patient does not think that they are related to the rape?

Targeted Physical Examination

- General exam: bruises, scratch marks, bite marks, and any pieces of evidence that the attacker may have left behind (e.g., clothing fibers, hairs, saliva, semen) that may help identify him
- Brief CNS, CVS, and RS exams

Case 57   Nicole Hitman is a 36-year-old woman who comes to the clinic with a history of recurrent spontaneous abortions.

Differential Diagnoses

1. Chromosomal abnormalities
2. TORCH infection (toxoplasmosis, other [congenital syphilis and viruses], rubella, cytomegalovirus, and herpes simplex virus)
3. Uterine anomalies
4. Hypothyroidism
5. Antiphospholipid antibody syndrome
6. Cervical incompetence
7. Chronic diseases

Investigations

1. Pelvic exam
2. Breast exam
3. Beta-human chorionic gonadotropin
4. Karyotype
5. TSH, T_3, T_4 levels
6. CBC with DC
7. Electrolytes
8. Hysterosalpingography

Red Flags

1. Diseases such as anemia, hypertension, or urinary tract infection can cause abortion.
2. Cervical incompetence leads to complications in the second trimester. Painless cervical dilation may lead to the delivery of a nonviable fetus.

Case 58   Sally Feeds is a 28-year-old woman with hematemesis.

Differential Diagnoses

1. Duodenal ulcer
2. Gastric ulcer
3. Erosive gastritis
4. Esophageal ulcer
5. Angiodysplasia
6. Mallory-Weiss tears

Investigations

1. CBC with DC
2. Electrolytes
3. EGD
4. Barium swallow examination
5. Nasogastric tube aspiration
6. Fecal occult blood test

7. Arteriogram
8. Blood typing and cross-matching

Red Flags

1. Alcohol abuse, liver diseases, and bleeding tendencies are red flags.
2. A history of warfarin, heparin, or aspirin use, or of vitamin K deficiency, or of von Willebrand's disease is a red flag.

Focused History

- What is the amount of blood lost?
- Is it frank blood or of coffee-ground appearance?
- Is melena present also?
- Any rectal urgency, straining, or pain with defecation?
- Ask about prior bleeding episodes, alcohol use, liver disease, coagulation disorders, NSAID history, history of radiation, recent surgery, aspirin intake.

Targeted Physical Examination

- General exam
- Examination of oral cavity
- Abdominal exam plus brief CVS and RS exams

Case 59   Jackie Dhan is a 36-year-old man complaining of itching.

Differential Diagnoses

1. Urticaria/angioedema
2. Food allergies
3. Medications
4. Infectious disease
5. Vasculitis
6. Idiopathic pruritus

Investigations

1. CBC with DC
2. Electrolytes
3. IgE levels
4. Liver function tests
5. Skin testing
6. TSH, T_3, T_4 levels

Red Flags

1. Urticaria: migratory, erythematous, raised, pruritic lesions that rarely persist more than 24 hours; 50% of patients also develop angioedema.
2. Anything can cause a rash, from food and insect bites to infectious processes.
3. Medications may be a part of life-threatening anaphylaxis. Adverse drug reactions include morbilliform rashes, serum sickness, fixed drug eruption (NSAIDs, sulfa drug),

photosensitivity, erythema multiforme, Stevens-Johnson syndrome, or even toxic epidermal necrolysis. Penicillin skin testing is available to detect the presence of persistent IgE antibody in those with penicillin allergy.

Focused History

- Location of the rash
- How the rash started initially
- Joint pains, fever, contacts with a similar rash, travel history, insect bites, allergies, recent medications

Targeted Physical Examination

- General exam
- Oral exam for mouth ulcers
- If there is pain in any joint, joint examination
- Brief CVS, RS, and abdominal exams

Case 60   Toby McDire is a 23-year-old man brought to the ED by paramedics. He was involved in a high-speed motor vehicle accident and complains of difficulty breathing.

Differential Diagnoses

1. Tension pneumothorax
2. Cardiac tamponade
3. Hypovolemia
4. Trauma to abdomen
5. Trauma to chest
6. Spinal cord injury
7. Intracranial hemorrhage

Investigations

1. Pelvic exam/rectal exam
2. Fasting blood sugar level
3. X-ray of cervical spine
4. Chest x-ray: portable AP and lateral views
5. CBC with DC, blood typing and cross-matching
6. ECG
7. Electrolytes
8. Blood alcohol level
9. US, diagnostic peritoneal lavage
10. CT of abdomen, head

Red Flags

1. Trauma to the abdomen poses the risk of splenic rupture, liver laceration, pelvic fractures, and any other viscous injury or perforation.
2. Trauma to the chest poses the risk of fracture of a rib, hemothorax, pulmonary contusion, air embolism, and flail chest.

Focused History

- Use mnemonic AMPLE:

  - ☐ Allergies
  - ☐ Medications
  - ☐ Past illness
  - ☐ Last meal
  - ☐ Events or environment related to injury

- What is the mechanism of injury (e.g., motor vehicle accident)?
  Were any of the six "Ss" involved: seizure, syncope, sugar (hypoglycemia), suicide, sleep, or sauce (alcohol)?
  Was penetrating trauma (e.g., bullets, knives, impaling object), a burn injury, or a cold injury involved?

Targeted Physical Examination

- General exam
- Mnemonic DR. ABCDEFGHI for trauma exam

Case 61   Adam Mandler, a 22-year-old medical student overly stressed by the USMLE Step 2-CS, ingested 30 tablets from an unlabeled bottle. He now wants to live, after a friend brought this book to his attention.

Differential Diagnoses

1. Acetaminophen poisoning
2. Digoxin poisoning
3. Beta-blocker poisoning
4. Lithium poisoning
5. Iron poisoning
6. Salicylate poisoning
7. Carbamazepine poisoning
8. Valproic acid poisoning
9. Theophylline poisoning

Investigations

1. Call the poison center.
2. Rectal exam, fecal occult blood test
3. CBC with DC, electrolytes
4. Urinalysis
5. Arterial blood gases
6. Serum toxicology screen, urine toxicology screen
7. Liver function tests
8. BUN, creatinine levels
9. ECG
10. Serum osmolarity, osmolar gap

Red Flags

1. The differential diagnosis lists the most common pill-induced poisonings.
2. Give support to the patient. Understand the reason behind the poisoning. Inform the patient that you will admit him to the hospital.
3. Each poison has its own specific signs and symptoms. Know the clinical features associated with each poison.
4. Up to 50% of all initial poisoning histories may be incorrect. Hence you must seek identification of the drug or drugs ingested.

Focused History

- Ask for supporting materials, such as the pill bottle.
- Specifically ask about the timing of the ingestion.
- Do a very brief time/place/orientation check and obtain a brief neurologic status history.

Targeted Physical Examination

- General exam
- Brief neurologic status exam, pupillary reaction to light
- Brief CVS and RS exams

Case 62   Kate Hoss is a thin 23-year-old woman who is on a crash diet because she thinks she is overweight.

Differential Diagnoses

1. Anorexia nervosa
2. Bulimia nervosa
3. Body dysmorphic disorder
4. Hyperthyroidism
5. Malabsorption syndrome
6. Substance abuse

Investigations

1. CBC with DC
2. Electrolytes
3. ECG
4. Urinalysis
5. Urine toxicology screen
6. TSH, T_3, T_4 levels
7. Stool for ova/cysts
8. Skin-fold thickness

Case 63 Melon Herren, a 27-year-old woman with a history of amenorrhea for the past 2 months, complains of nausea and vomiting.

Differential Diagnoses

1. Normal pregnancy
2. Ectopic pregnancy
3. Pseudocyesis
4. Molar pregnancy
5. Twin pregnancy
6. High-risk pregnancy

Investigations

1. Pelvic exam, breast exam
2. Beta-human chorionic gonadotropin level
3. Pap smear
4. Urinalysis
5. CBC with DC
6. ABO and Rh typing
7. TORCH screen
8. Hepatitis B and HIV screening
9. US of abdomen

Red Flags

1. Amenorrhea and morning sickness with nausea and vomiting are the classic symptoms of pregnancy. Hogar's sign (softening and thinning of the lower uterine segment), Chadwick's sign (a bluish discoloration of the vaginal and vulva walls), linea nigra, melasma (mask of pregnancy), and weight gain are also signs of pregnancy. The patient may also complain of backache, heartburn, and frequent urination.
2. Hypertension, diabetes, heart disease, Rh incompatibility, hydatidiform mole, and TORCH injections should be actively sought and ruled out.
3. Advise folate therapy to prevent neural tube defects.
4. Listen for fetal heart tones. Evaluate uterine size for size/dates discrepancy.

Focused History

- Ask about last menstrual period. Obtain a complete obstetric/gynecologic history, history of rubella immunization, CVS problems, sleep and appetite, history of medication/drug use or abuse, history of STDs.

Targeted Physical Examination

- General exam
- Brief CVS and RS exams
- Complete examination of the abdomen

Case 64   Russell Browe, a 32-year-old man, is brought to the clinic by his wife because he hit his neighbor and took away his neighbor's cat. He put the cat in the microwave because "the voice from Uranus told me to." He complains that he hears voices that tell him what to do.

Differential Diagnoses

1. Schizophrenia, paranoid type
2. Delusional disorder
3. Brief psychotic disorder
4. Paranoid personality disorder
5. Substance-induced psychotic disorder

Investigations

1. CBC with DC
2. Electrolytes
3. Urinalysis
4. Fasting blood sugar level
5. Urine toxicology screen
6. Serum toxicology screen

Red Flags

1. Schizophrenia: delusions, hallucinations, disorganized speech or behavior, negative symptoms, as well as preoccupation with delusions/hallucinations, typically of grandiosity or persecution. The patient must have significant social or occupational dysfunction.
2. Delusional disorder: nonbizarre delusions, with no marked deterioration in level of functioning.
3. Brief psychotic disorder: any type of schizophrenia symptoms that last at least 1 day but less than 1 month.
4. Positive symptoms of schizophrenia: delusions, hallucinations, disorganized speech/thinking, catatonic behaviors.
5. Negative symptoms of schizophrenia: affective flattening, alogia or poverty of speech, avolition.
6. Other symptoms sometimes present in schizophrenia but not often enough to be definitional alone include affect inappropriate to the situation or stimuli, unusual motor behavior (pacing, rocking), depersonalization, derealization, and somatic preoccupations.

Focused History

- Use the mnemonic CASE THIS IF MORPHINE JOKE, then PMH.

Targeted Physical Examination

- General exam
- Brief CVS and RS exams

Case 65   Jennifer Fairy, a 47-year-old disheveled woman, is brought to the ED by her husband of 22 years. He claims that she has maxed out her credit cards and has spent their life savings by checking into a suite at the Ritz and leasing a Ferrari; also, she has left a message at the White House to call back urgently. She arranged a meeting with real estate agents to purchase a palatial home in the Hamptons.

Differential Diagnoses

1. Bipolar I disorder
2. Substance-induced mood disorder
3. Cyclothymic disorder
4. Hyperthyroidism
5. Psychotic disorder

Investigations

1. CBC with DC
2. Electrolytes
3. TSH, T_3, T_4 levels
4. Urinalysis
5. Urine toxicology screen
6. Serum toxicology screen

Red Flags

1. Bipolar I disorder: one manic episode or mixed manic episode with mood disturbances, increased self-esteem, grandiosity, decreased sleep, flight of ideas, excessive involvement in high-risk pleasurable activities.
2. Cyclothymic disorder: symptoms present for at least 2 years. Numerous alternating hypomanic and depressed mood episodes.

Focused History

- Use the mnemonic CASE THIS IF MORPHINE JOKE, then PMH.

Targeted Physical Examination

- General exam
- Brief CVS and RS exams

9

35 Practice Cases

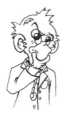

Write your answers to these practice cases. Then go to Chapter 10, page 121, to check your answers.

Case 1: Paris Fulton, a 22-year-old woman with a history of acne

Case 2: Heath Richards, a 44-year-old man with a history of blood in his urine for the past 2 days

Case 3: Flint Eastwood, a 62-year-old man complaining of shortness of breath

Case 4: Beryl Sweep, a 32-year-old woman brought to the ED by her husband, with whom she has had problems

Case 5: Helen DeGeneres, a 55-year-old woman complaining of progressive hearing loss

Case 6: Bony Hopkins, a 45-year-old man worried that his wife wants a divorce because of his loud snoring

Case 7: David Marquette, a 22-year-old man with knee pain, back pain, and acute pleuritic chest pain

Case 8: Julie Roberta, a 40-year-old woman with a lump in her left breast

Case 9: Teal Armstrong, a 25-year-old man who wants to be an astronaut

Case 10: Tom Harly, a 45-year-old man with swollen glands in his neck

Case 11: Russell Simon, a 44-year-old man with pain in his right leg for the past 2 weeks

Case 12: Kimora Simon, a 65-year-old woman with headache and decreased vision in her right eye for the past 2 days

Case 13: Dick Lacey, a 33-year-old man with progressive altered mental status for the past 4 months

Case 14: Rob Snow, a 37-year-old man with acute shortness of breath

Case 15: Joey Soprano, a 35-year-old man with a history of heroin abuse

Case 16: Kelly Larkson, a 27-year-old woman who wants to quit smoking

Case 17: Bryan Neilly, a 68-year-old man complaining of diarrhea and weight loss for more than 1 year

Case 18: Victory Beckman, a 24-year-old woman complaining of red eyes for the past 4 days

Case 19: Benvenuto Bellini, a 33-year-old man with a genital ulcer

Case 20: Doll Flanders, a 27-year-old woman with a history of multiple sexual partners and seizures for the past 4 hours

Case 21: Sarah Justin Barker, a 45-year-old woman with a history of mitral valve prolapse and complaints of palpitations

Case 22: Jorge Berns, a 65-year-old man with lower left quadrant pain and fever for 1 day

Case 23: Mike Ditza, a 62-year-old man with a history of hypertension and complaints of shortness of breath

Case 24: B.D. Sting, a 73-year-old African American with a history of hypertension and complaints of loss of consciousness for 1 hour

Case 25: Dunstin Offman, a 60-year-old hypervigilant man with clouding of consciousness

Case 26: Kylie Ninogue, a mother who complains that her 1-year-old son has a discharge from his left ear and fever for the past 2 days

Case 27: Jane Bustle, an 18-year-old woman worried that her breasts are too large

Case 28: Jerry Mall, a 46-year-old woman with complaints of an aching, pricking, and tingling sensation in her right hand

Case 29: Heather Raham, a 40-year-old woman complaining of abdominal fullness for the past 3 months

Case 30: Jake Black, a 38-year-old man with a history of hypertension and complaints of swelling in his legs

Case 31: Gary Goldman, a 50-year-old man with no urine output for the past 2 days

Case 32: Tank O'Mara, a 47-year-old man with a history of hypertension, type 2 diabetes, and chronic alcoholism and complaints of shortness of breath and fever

Case 33: Ricky Bilboa, a 32-year-old boxer with AIDS and complaints of cough and chest pain for the past 2 days

Case 34: Leigh Stemick, a 62-year-old woman with a history of hypertension and chest pain for the past 6 hours

Case 35: Ernie Lemonway, a 43-year-old man with a history of alcoholism and current attempts to withdraw

Bonus Case: Mr. Alzheimer Lewis, a 78-year-old man with progressive memory loss

---

Case 1   Paris Fulton is a 22-year-old woman with a history of acne. She presents with acne for the past 6 months on her face. She says she has tried every available over-the-counter medication and nothing seems to work.

Differential Diagnoses

1.
2.
3.
4.
5.

Investigations

1.
2.
3.
4.
5.

Case 2   Heath Richards is a 44-year-old man with a history of blood in his urine for the past 2 days.

Differential Diagnoses

1.
2.
3.
4.
5.

Investigations

1.
2.
3.
4.
5

Case 3   Flint Eastwood is a 62-year-old man complaining of shortness of breath. His cardiovascular examination shows a 3/6 systolic murmur.

Differential Diagnoses

1.
2.
3.
4
5.

Investigations

1.
2.
3.
4.
5.

Case 4   Beryl Sweep is a 32-year-old woman who was brought to the ED by her husband, with whom she has had problems. Her husband indicates that he found her sweating profusely and that she may have taken something orally. Her electrolytes indicate an increase in the anion gap.

Differential Diagnoses

1.
2.
3.
4.
5.

Investigations

1.
2.
3.
4.
5.

Case 5   Helen DeGeneres is a 55-year-old woman complaining that she cannot listen to her new I-Pod. She states that she has noticed progressive hearing loss for the past 6 months.

Differential Diagnoses

1.
2.
3.
4.
5.

Investigations

1.
2.
3.
4.
5.

Case 6   Bony Hopkins is a 45-year-old man worried that his wife wants a divorce. He states that his wife does not like him any more because he snores very loudly.

Differential Diagnoses

1.
2.
3.
4.
5.

Investigations

1.
2.
3.
4.
5.

Case 7   David Marquette is a 22-year-old man with knee pain, back pain, and acute pleuritic chest pain. He states that he has sickle cells in his blood.

Differential Diagnoses

1.
2.
3.
4.
5.

Investigations

1.
2.
3.
4.
5.

Case 8   Julie Roberta is a 40-year-old woman with a lump in her left breast. She says that she noticed it 2 weeks ago when she was hit by a ball in the same area.

Differential Diagnoses

1.
2.
3.
4.
5.

Investigations

1.
2.
3.
4.
5.

Case 9   Teal Amstrong is a 25-year-old man who wants to be an astronaut. He is being screened by NASA for a physical examination. (They will require you to perform specific tests as a pre-employment screening.)

Case 10   Tom Harly is a 45-year-old man with swollen glands in his neck (lymphadenopathy).

Differential Diagnoses

1.
2.
3.
4.
5.

Investigations

1.
2.
3.
4.
5.

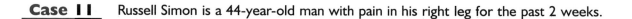

Case 11   Russell Simon is a 44-year-old man with pain in his right leg for the past 2 weeks.

Differential Diagnoses

1.
2.
3.
4.
5.

Investigations

1.
2.
3.
4.
5.

Case 12   Kimora Simon is a 65-year-old woman with headache and decreased vision in her right eye for the past 2 days.

Differential Diagnoses

1.
2.
3.
4.
5.

Investigations

1.
2.
3.
4.
5.

Case 13   Dick Lacey is a 33-year-old man with progressive altered mental status for the past 4 months.

Differential Diagnoses

1.
2.
3.
4.
5.

Investigations

1.
2.
3.
4.
5.

Case 14   Rob Snow is a 37-year-old man with acute shortness of breath. On examination he has bilateral wheezes present in his chest.

Differential Diagnoses

1.
2.
3.
4.
5.

Investigations

1.
2.
3.
4.
5.

Case 15   Joey Soprano is a 35-year-old man with a history of heroin abuse. He states that he wants a prescription for codeine for chronic pain in his little finger.

Differential Diagnoses

1.
2.
3.
4.
5.

Investigations

1.
2.
3.
4.
5.

Case 16   Kelly Larkson is a 27-year-old woman worried that no man will go on a date with her because she is unable to quit smoking.

Case 17   Bryan Neilly is a 68-year-old man complaining of diarrhea and weight loss for more than 1 year.

Differential Diagnoses

1.
2.
3.
4.
5.

Investigations

1.
2.
3.
4.
5.

Case 18   Victory Beckman is a 24-year-old woman complaining of red eyes for the past 4 days.

Differential Diagnoses

1.
2.
3.
4.
5.

Investigations

1.
2.
3.
4.
5.

Case 19   Benventuo Bellini is a 33-year-old man with a genital ulcer.

Differential Diagnoses

1.
2.
3.
4.
5.

Investigations

1.
2.
3.
4.
5.

Case 20 Doll Flanders is a 27-year-old woman with a history of multiple sexual partners. She presents to the ED with a seizure for 4 hours prior to admission. On examination, she has a right facial droop.

Differential Diagnoses

1.
2.
3.
4.
5.

Investigations

1.
2.
3.
4.
5.

Case 21 Sarah Justin Barker is a 45-year-old woman with a history of mitral valve prolapse. She complains of palpitations off and on for the past 2 years. She has seen many doctors and states that no one can treat her.

Differential Diagnoses

1.
2.
3.
4.
5.

Investigations

1.
2.
3.
4.
5.

Case 22   Jorge Berns is a 65-year-old man with lower left quadrant pain and fever for 1 day.

Differential Diagnoses

1.
2.
3.
4.
5.

Investigations

1.
2.
3.
4.
5.

Case 23   Mike Ditza is a 62-year-old man with a history of hypertension. He complains of shortness of breath since yesterday.

Differential Diagnoses

1.
2.
3.
4.
5.

Investigations

1.
2.
3.
4.
5.

Case 24   B.D. Sting is a 73-year-old African-American man with a history of hypertension. He complains of loss of consciousness for 1 hour a few days ago.

Differential Diagnoses

1.
2.
3.
4.
5.

Investigations

1.
2.
3.
4.
5.

Case 25   Dunstin Offman is a 60-year-old hypervigilant man with clouding of consciousness.

Differential Diagnoses

1.
2.
3.
4.
5.

Investigations

1.
2.
3.
4.
5.

Case 26   Kylie Ninogue is the mother of a 1-year-old boy. She complains that her son has a discharge from his left ear and fever for the past 2 days.

Differential Diagnoses

1.
2.
3.
4.
5.

Investigations

1.
2.
3.
4.
5.

Case 27   Jane Bustle is an 18-year-old woman worried that her breasts are too large.

Differential Diagnoses

1.
2.
3.
4.
5.

Investigations

1.
2.
3.
4.
5.

Case 28 Jerry Mall is a 46-year-old woman with complaints of an aching, pricking, and tingling sensation of pins and needles in her right hand.

Differential Diagnoses

1.
2.
3.
4.
5.

Investigations

1.
2.
3.
4.
5.

Case 29 Heather Raham is a 40-year-old woman complaining of abdominal fullness for the past 3 months.

Differential Diagnoses

1.
2.
3.
4.
5.

Investigations

1.
2.
3.
4.
5.

Case 30   Jake Black is a 38-year-old man with a history of complaints of swelling in his legs. He also has a history of hypertension for the past 8 years.

Differential Diagnoses

1.
2.
3.
4.
5.

Investigations

1.
2.
3.
4.
5.

Case 31   Gary Goldman is a 50-year-old man with no urine output for the past 2 days.

Differential Diagnoses

1.
2.
3.
4.
5.

Investigations

1.
2.
3.
4.
5.

Case 32   Tank O'Mara is a 47-year-old man with a history of hypertension for the past 17 years, type 2 diabetes mellitus for the past 5 years, and chronic alcoholism for the past 27 years. He complains of shortness of breath and fever for the past 2 days.

Differential Diagnoses

1.
2.
3.
4.
5.

Investigations

1.
2.
3.
4.
5.

Case 33   Ricky Bilboa is a 32-year-old boxer with AIDS. He complains of cough and pain on the right side of his chest for the past 2 days.

Differential Diagnoses

1.
2.
3.
4.
5.

Investigations

1.
2.
3.
4.
5.

Case 34   Leigh Stemick is a 62-year-old woman with a history of hypertension. She has an abnormal ECG and an increase in serum potassium levels on routine screening. She has had pain in her chest for the past 6 hours.

Differential Diagnoses

1.
2.
3.
4.
5.

Investigations

1.
2.
3.
4.
5.

Case 35   Ernie Lemonway is a 43-year-old man with a history of alcoholism for the past 13 years. He recently has been trying to quit cold turkey but has been experimenting with different drugs to cope with the problems of withdrawal. He presents to your clinic with neck rigidity and fever.

Differential Diagnoses

1.
2.
3.
4.
5.

Investigations

1.
2.
3.
4.
5.

Bonus Case   Mr. Alzheimer Lewis is a 78-year-old man with progressive memory loss. Do a Mini-Mental Status Exam on the sheet provided.

10

ANSWERS FOR THE 35 PRACTICE CASES

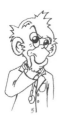

Case 1   **Differential Diagnoses**

1. Acne
2. Rosacea
3. Folliculitis
4. Milia
5. Steroid acne
6. Contact dermatitis
7. Miliaria
8. Seborrheic dermatitis

Investigations

1. CBC with DC
2. BMP
3. Liver function tests
4. Pregnancy test
5. Serum lipid profile

Red Flags

1. Acne is a very common condition. Many cases are resistant to over-the-counter medications. You may need to refer the patient to a dermatologist.

Case 2   **Differential Diagnoses**

1. Urinary tract infection, pyelonephritis
2. Benign prostatic hypertrophy
3. Glomerular disease
4. Hypersensitivity reaction—vascular disease
5. Renal infarction
6. Renal cell carcinoma
7. Nephrolithiasis

8. Coagulation abnormalities
9. Trauma
10. Drug toxicity

Investigations

1. Pelvic and rectal exam
2. Urinalysis: dipstick, microscopic
3. Urine culture
4. X-ray of kidney, ureter, bladder (KUB)
5. IV urography
6. CT/MRI
7. Cystoscopy
8. Renal angiogram

 ### Red Flags

1. Carcinoma is associated with advanced age.
2. Cyclophosphamide is associated with hemorrhagic cystitis.
3. Moderate to severe trauma from the loin to the groin area, as well as in the suprapubic area, can cause hematuria.
4. Inform the patient that you will discuss the case further with a nephrologist or urologist.

Case 3   ### Differential Diagnoses

1. Acute pulmonary edema
2. Acute exacerbation of congestive heart failure
3. Arrhythmia
4. Ischemia
5. Myocardial infarction
6. Valve rupture
7. Papillary muscle rupture
8. Pneumonia
9. Chronic obstructive pulmonary disease
10. Asthma

Investigations

1. CBC with DC
2. BMP
3. ECG
4. Chest x-ray
5. Arterial blood gases
6. Cardiac enzymes
7. Pulse oximetry
8. Telemetry
9. Echocardiography

 ### Red Flags

1. Examine the lower extremities for edema.
2. Counsel about the adverse effects of smoking.
3. Because of the age of the patient, a history detailing the activities of daily living should not be overlooked.

Case 4   **Differential Diagnoses**

1. Lactic acidosis
2. Methanol
3. Uremia
4. Diabetic ketoacidosis
5. Paraldehyde poisoning
6. Isoniazid poisoning
7. Ethanol poisoning
8. Salicylate poisoning

Investigations

1. Fingerstick glucose test
2. CBC with DC
3. Electrolytes
4. Urinalysis with ketones
5. Serum for ketones
6. Blood sugar levels
7. Urine toxicology screen

 Red Flags

1. Remember the mnemonic for metabolic acidosis (Lovely MUD PIES).

Case 5   **Differential Diagnoses**

1. Presbycusis
2. Noise-induced hearing loss
3. Hypercoagulable states
4. Ménière's disease
5. Acoustic neuroma
6. Tertiary syphilis
7. Perilymphatic fistula
8. Trauma
9. Hypothyroidism
10. Diabetes mellitus

Investigations

1. CBC with DC
2. ESR
3. TSH, T_3, T_4 levels
4. Urinalysis
5. Serum glucose
6. Respiratory function tests
7. Syphilis serology
8. Lyme titer
9. MRI of the head at the internal auditory canal

Red Flags

1. You must be able to distinguish between conductive and sensorineural deafness.
2. Remember the triad for Ménière's disease: deafness, vertigo, and tinnitus.
3. The patient's hearing loss may be situation-dependent. The patient may hear normally in a quiet room but have problems in a noisy environment.
4. If the patient speaks loudly, the diagnosis leans toward presbycusis.
5. Otoscopy and Weber's and Rinne's tests must be performed.

Case 6   Differential Diagnoses

1. Obstructive sleep apnea
2. Nasal obstruction
3. Adenoidal or tonsillar hypertrophy
4. Nocturnal hypoventilation syndrome
5. Scoliosis
6. Macroglossia
7. Acromegaly
8. Hypothyroidism
9. Vocal cord paralysis

Investigations

1. EEG
2. Electro-oculogram
3. Electromyelogram
4. Overnight pulse-oximetry
5. End-tidal CO_2 pressure
6. Inductance plethysmography
7. Microphone assessment of snoring
8. Thermistor

 Red Flags

1. Examine the oral and nasal cavity.
2. Obesity is a common cause of obstructive sleep apnea.
3. Look for a history of alcoholism, smoking, morning headaches, impaired concentration, and awakening unrefreshed.

Case 7   Differential Diagnoses

1. Vaso-occlusive crisis
2. Pulmonary infarction
3. Pneumonia
4. Osteomyelitis
5. Cholecystitis
6. Pancreatitis
7. Pericarditis
8. Trauma

Investigations

1. CBC with DC
2. Peripheral smear
3. Serum bilirubin
4. Urinalysis
5. Airway, breathing, and circulation
6. Chest x-ray: PA and lateral views
7. ECG
8. Hemoglobin electrophoresis

Red Flags

1. Dehydration, hypoxia, and infection predispose a patient with sickle cell anemia to a vaso-occlusive crisis.
2. A history of hemolysis and hematuria may be present.
3. Infections with encapsulated organisms are common.
4. Inform the patient that you will give pain medications immediately after your encounter.

Case 8   ### Differential Diagnoses

1. Fibroadenoma
2. Benign breast mass
3. Breast cyst
4. Breast cancer
5. Breast abscess
6. Trauma

Investigations

1. Breast examination
2. CBC with DC
3. Mammogram
4. Ultrasonography
5. Breast cyst aspiration
6. Cytology of any discharge

Red Flags

1. A postmenopausal, asymmetrical mass is highly suspect for breast cancer.
2. A premenopausal breast mass may be benign, but malignancy must be ruled out.
3. Mammograms are recommended for all women older than 30 years who are not lactating.
4. Inform the patient that a breast examination is necessary and will be done at a later time with another woman present.

Case 9   For this case of pre-employment screening a list of tasks will be presented to you on the doorway information (perform cardiovascular, respiratory, and visual examinations). Inside the examination room, the SP will hand you a form with the list of tasks on it. You are required to perform only the tasks on the list. You will probably not be required to devise a differential diagnosis or a list of investigations. The only write-up may be filling out the form that the SP hands you.

Case 10   Differential Diagnoses

1. Hematological disorder
2. Infections: viral, bacterial, fungal, TB
3. Immunological disorder: rheumatoid arthritis, systemic lupus erythematosus
4. Connective tissue disease
5. Chronic lymphocytic leukemia
6. Unknown lipid storage disease
7. Primary neoplasm
8. Secondary neoplasm
9. Sarcoidosis

Investigations

1. CBC with DC
2. Chest x-ray
3. Lactate dehydrogenase level
4. Serology: viral (Epstein-Barr virus, cytomegalovirus, HIV), bacterial (TB, syphilis)
5. Antinuclear antibody test
6. TSH level
7. CT scan
8. Lymph node biopsy
9. Bone marrow biopsy

Red Flags

1. Use of the mnemonic HIICCUPSS will help you with the differential diagnosis.
2. Enlargment of the left supraclavicular lymph node indicates metastasis from the stomach or pancreas.
3. Use of drugs such as phenytoin and antithyroid medications must be ruled out.
4. A malignancy search with risk factors must be undertaken.

Case 11   Differential Diagnoses

1. Deep venous thrombosis
2. Intermittent claudication (peripheral vascular disease)
3. Arterial thromboembolism
4. Lumber canal stenosis
5. Peripheral neuropathy
6. Night cramps
7. Ligament strain
8. Cellulitis
9. Muscle or tendon strain

Investigations

1. CBC with DC
2. BMP
3. Doppler study of the left leg
4. X-ray of the left leg: PA and lateral views

5. X-ray of the lumbar spine
6. ESR

Red Flags

1. Pain that is position-related strongly suggests spinal cord stenosis.
2. Any history of alcohol use or abnormal blood glucose can lead to peripheral neuropathy.

Case 12   Differential Diagnoses

1. Temporal arteritis
2. Migraine headache
3. Tension headache
4. Cluster headache
5. Trauma
6. Subarachnoid hemorrhage
7. Malignancy
8. Glaucoma
9. Sinusitis

Investigations

1. ESR
2. C-reactive protein
3. CBC with DC
4. Lumbar puncture
5. X-ray: Waters' view
6. Tonometry
7. CT of head
8. Temporal artery biopsy

Red Flags

1. Temporal arteritis typically begins after age 50 in women. It is associated with polymyalgia rheumatica—proximal limb girdle pain.

Case 13   Differential Diagnoses

1. Infection
2. Withdrawal
3. Acute metabolic causes
4. Trauma
5. CNS causes
6. Hypoxia
7. Deficiencies (nutritional)
8. Endocrine
9. Acute vascular causes

10. Toxins/drugs
11. Heavy metals

Investigations

1. CBC with DC
2. CMP
3. ESR, C-reactive protein
4. Pulse oximetry
5. Urine toxicology screen
6. Alcohol levels
7. TSH, T_3, T_4 levels
8. CT/MRI
9. Serum levels of vitamin B_{12}
10. Lead levels

Red Flags

1. The mnemonic I WATCH DEATH can be helpful.

Case 14   Differential Diagnoses

1. Acute asthma exacerbation
2. Foreign body obstruction
3. Pneumonia
4. Trauma
5. Spontaneous pneumothorax
6. Acute congestive heart failure
7. Bacterial pneumonia

Investigations

1. CBC with DC
2. BMP
3. Chest x-ray: PA and lateral views
4. Arterial blood gases
5. Peak flow
6. Sputum Gram stain and culture
7. Blood culture
8. Pulmonary function tests/spirometry
9. Diffusion study

Red Flags

1. Shortness of breath + diffuse wheezing = asthma.
2. Shortness of breath + cough + absence of air entry on affected side = spontaneous pneumothorax.

Case 15 **Differential Diagnoses**

1. Drug abuse
2. Drug withdrawal
3. Trauma
4. HIV
5. Hepatitis
6. Fracture/dislocation

Investigations

1. CBC with DC
2. BMP
3. Urine toxicology screen
4. Serum toxicology screen
5. X-ray: AP and lateral views
6. ELISA
7. Hepatitis panel

 Red Flags

1. Counsel patient about the adverse effects of drug abuse.
2. Patient consent is required for an ELISA. You must indicate why the patient is at higher risk for HIV.

Case 16 ■ You must reassure the patient that you can help her quit smoking if she so desires.
 ■ Emphasize positive outcomes, such as:

  ☐ Decreased cancer risks: lung, larynx, oral cavity, esophagus, bladder, cervix
  ☐ Decreased risk of MI, stroke, peripheral vascular disease
  ☐ Improved sexual performance

 ■ Assist in the effort.
 ■ Tell the patient to:

  ☐ Set a quit date.
  ☐ Dispose of all tobacco products and ashtrays.
  ☐ Try going cold turkey, which is the best method.

 ■ Reassure the patient that you will help by providing self-help materials, nicotine patches, and follow-up in person or by telephone.
 ■ Give her the option of attending a smoking cessation clinic.

Case 17 **Differential Diagnoses**

1. Colon cancer
2. Zollinger-Ellison syndrome
3. Irritable bowel syndrome
4. Inflammatory bowel disease
5. Hyperthyroidism

6. Malabsorption
7. HIV
8. Giardiasis/amebiasis

Investigations

1. CBC with DC
2. BMP
3. Colonoscopy/sigmoidoscopy
4. Stool culture
5. Fecal leukocyte count
6. TSH level
7. Upper GI series
8. Serum gastrin levels

Red Flags

1. Remember the age group for colon cancer screening.
2. The travel history is also very important. Recent travel to Mexico or to any developing nation increases the risk of infectious diarrhea.
3. A history of repeated peptic ulcers in the presence of pharmacologic treatment, along with watery diarrhea, suggests Zollinger-Ellison syndrome.

Case 18   ## Differential Diagnoses

1. Infectious conjunctivitis
2. Allergic conjunctivitis
3. Acute glaucoma
5. Iritis
6. Keratitis
7. Trauma
8. Iridocyclitis
9. Acute uveitis

Investigations

1. CBC with DC
2. Tonometry
3. Giemsa stain of conjunctival scrapings
4. Cytology of conjunctival scrapings
5. Slit lamp examination

Red Flags

1. An ophthalmoscopic examination is required.
2. Extreme pain + blurred vision + red eye + steamy cornea + pupil dilated + moderately non-reactive to light = acute glaucoma.

Case 19   **Differential Diagnoses**

1. Chancroid
2. Syphilitic chancre
3. Granuloma inguinale
4. Herpes simplex
5. Lymphogranuloma venereum
6. Hepatitis B
7. HIV

Investigations

1. CBC with DC
2. BMP
3. VDRL test for syphilis
4. *Chlamydia* testing
5. Gram stain
6. Dark-field microscopy
7. Culture of scraping

Red Flags

1. Soft chancre + painful = chancroid.
2. Hard chancre + painless = syphilis.

Case 20   **Differential Diagnoses**

1. Seizure with Todd's paralysis
2. Stroke with seizure
3. Brain tumor
4. Brain abscess
5. Arteriovenous malformation
6. Hyponatremia
7. Hypernatremia
8. Psychosis

Investigations

1. CBC with DC
2. BMP
3. Urine toxicology screen
4. CT with/without contrast
5. Chest x-ray
6. Urinalysis
7. Hepatitis B screening
8. ELISA

Red Flags

1. Multiple sexual partners put her at risk for HIV. Consent must be obtained for HIV testing. Consider a differential diagnosis of toxoplasmosis versus CNS lymphoma.

Case 21 **Differential Diagnoses**

1. Hyperthyroidism
2. Panic disorder
3. Supraventricular tachycardia
4. Generalized anxiety disorder
5. Pheochromocytoma
6. Substance abuse
7. Hypochondriasis

Investigations

1. ECG
2. TSH, T_3, T_4 levels
3. CBC with DC
4. Electrolytes
5. Blood culture
6. Urine vanillylmandelic acid level
7. Urine and serum toxicology screen
8. Blood glucose level

Red Flags

1. Episodic hypertension and headache are common presentations of pheochromocytoma.
2. In patients with mitral valve prolapse, one should rule out associated pathologies, such as diverticula of the colon, hepatic cysts, and polycystic kidney disease.

Case 22 **Differential Diagnoses**

1. Diverticulitis
2. Appendicitis
3. Peritonitis
4. Colon cancer
5. Colon perforation
6. Pyelonephritis
7. Left lower lobe pneumonia

Investigations

1. Rectal exam
2. CBC with DC
3. Urinalysis
4. BMP
5. Chest x-ray
6. X-ray of the abdomen
7. CT of the abdomen
8. Sigmoidoscopy/colonoscopy
9. Stool cultures
10. Ultrasonography of the abdomen

Red Flags

1. Diverticulitis can lead to perforation.
2. Remember the criteria for colon cancer screening. At the age of 50, an annual digital rectal exam and occult blood test of stool are recommended, as well as a colonoscopy every 3–5 years.

Case 23   Differential Diagnoses

1. Acute exacerbation of congestive heart failure
2. MI
3. Bronchitis
4. Pneumonia
5. Pneumothorax
6. Asthma
7. Pulmonary embolism

Investigations

1. CBC with DC
2. BMP
3. Brain natriuretic peptide
4. Chest x-ray
5. ECG
6. Echocardiography
7. Arterial blood gases
8. Pulse oximetry
9. V/Q scan
10. Spiral CT

Red Flags

1. If fever is present, the diagnosis leans toward pneumonia.
2. If fever is absent, think of asthma and bronchitis.
3. Remember that in atypical presentations of MI, pain can be absent. But the possibility of MI should always be ruled out.

Case 24   Differential Diagnoses

1. Transient ischemic attack
2. Stroke
3. Carotid occlusion
4. Hemorrhage
5. Hypertensive encephalopathy
6. Meningitis
7. Metastasis to brain

Investigations

1. CBC with DC
2. BMP
3. Doppler study of carotid vessels
4. CT scan of the head
5. Echocardiography
6. Lumbar puncture
7. ECG
8. Carotid angiography
9. MR angiography
10. Blood culture

Red Flags

1. With a history of atrial fibrillation or any other type of arrhythmia, an ECG should always be obtained.
2. Remember that MRI is better than CT for almost everything except blood. If you suspect intracranial hemorrhage, always do a plain CT study first.
3. Ask about any slurred speech or transient aphasia in the history.
4. Ask about any symptoms of vertigo, nausea, vomiting, tinnitus, and visual loss.
5. Drop attacks are sudden loss of postural tone in all four extremities.
6. Try to differentiate between carotid artery and vertebrobasilar artery syndrome.
7. Remember the risk factors for stroke: hypertension, smoking, obesity, hyperlipidemia, increased age, diabetes mellitus type 2, and homocystinuria.

Case 25   Differential Diagnoses

1. Infection
2. Intoxication
3. Ischemic/hemorrhagic stroke
4. Trauma
5. Electrolyte imbalance
6. Hypertensive encephalopathy
7. Hypoglycemia
8. Hepatic encephalopathy
9. Schizophrenia
10. Psychosis

Investigations

1. Pulse oximetry
2. BMP
3. CBC with DC
4. Urine toxicology screen
5. Urinalysis
6. Lumbar puncture
7. CT/MRI
8. Liver function tests

Red Flags

1. A proper psychiatric history is a must. Remember to perform a Mini-Mental Status Examination.

Case 26   Differential Diagnoses

1. Otitis media
2. Otitis interna
3. Otitis externa
4. Perforated tympanic membrane
5. Cerebral encephalitis
6. CSF otorrhea

Investigations

1. Otoscopy
2. CBC with DC
3. BMP
4. X-ray: Waters' view
5. Tympanocentesis
6. Culture of discharge
7. Blood culture

Red Flags

1. Otitis media is a common diagnosis in the neonatal and pediatric age group.
2. In a typical case the presentation includes otalgia, aural pressure, decreased hearing, fever, and discharge from ear.
3. The three most common bacterial causes of otitis media are *Streptococcus pneumoniae*, *Moxarella catarrhalis*, and *Hemophilus influenzae*.

Case 27   Differential Diagnoses

1. Normal puberty
2. Klinefelter's syndrome
3. Secondary hypogonadism
4. Estrogen-producing tumors
5. Liver failure
6. Renal failure
7. Drugs
8. Cushing's syndrome

Investigations

1. Testosterone level
2. Follicle-stimulating hormone, luteinizing hormone levels
3. Liver function tests
4. Thyroid functions tests
5. DHEAS level
6. Prolactin level
7. Beta-human chorionic gonadotropin level
8. Ultrasonography of abdomen and groin
9. CT of abdomen
10. Karyotype

Red Flags

1. A specific drug history must be taken. The use of spironolactone, cimetidine, digoxin, and even marijuana can cause gynecomastia and engorgement of breast.

Case 28

Differential Diagnoses

1. Carpal tunnel syndrome
2. Diabetes mellitus
3. Vitamin B_{12} deficiency
4. Chronic renal failure
5. Drugs
6. Hypoparathyroidism
7. Guillain-Barré syndrome
8. Multiple sclerosis

Investigations

1. Arterial blood gases
2. Serum calcium
3. Serum parathyroid hormone
4. Blood glucose, hemoglobin 1ac
5. Serum magnesium
6. Vitamin B_{12} level
7. Nerve conduction studies
8. TSH, T_3, T_4 levels

Red Flags

1. Determine whether the paresthesia is persistent or transient.
2. If the paresthesia is persistent along a single nerve, think of neuralgia paresthetica.
3. Acute hypocalcemia can cause perioral paresthesia.
4. Metronidazole, nitrofurantoin, isoniazid, and vinca alkaloids are neurotoxic drugs.

Case 29

Differential Diagnoses

1. Malignancy
2. Cirrhosis
3. Portal hypertension
4. Hypoproteinemia
5. Right heart failure
6. Obesity
7. Fecal impaction
8. Flatus

Investigations

1. CBC with DC
2. BMP
3. Liver function tests
4. Ultrasonography of the abdomen
5. CT of the abdomen
6. Serum albumin concentration
7. Ascitic tap
8. X-ray of the abdomen

Red Flags

1. Fat, fluid, feces, flatus, fetus, forty, and full bladder are the seven Fs that can cause abdominal distention.
2. If fever is present, suspect peritonitis.
3. On the abdominal examination, look for free fluid in the abdomen. Look for shifting dullness, a fluid thrill on percussion, and any signs of chronic liver disease, lymphadenopathy, or edema, as well as elevated jugular venous pressure.

Case 30   Differential Diagnoses

1. Deep vein thrombosis
2. Cellulitis
3. Lymphatic obstruction
4. Right ventricular failure
5. Congestive heart failure
6. Nephrotic syndrome
7. Drugs
8. Immobility
9. Malnutrition

Investigations

1. CBC with DC
2. Doppler study of left leg
3. Liver function tests
4. Urine dipstick test
5. Chest x-ray
6. ECG
7. Urine protein/creatine ratio
8. Echocardiography
9. Contrast venography

Red Flags

1. Swollen legs are common in patients with cardiac, renal, or hepatic conditions.
2. Determine whether the swelling is unilateral or bilateral.
3. Questions that must be answered are:

   ☐ Does the swelling pit with digital pressure?
   ☐ Is the swelling associated with breathlessness?
   ☐ Is ascites present?

Case 31   Differential Diagnoses

1. Benign prostatic hypertrophy
2. Pelvic mass
3. Drugs
4. Spinal cord lesions
5. Tumor

6. Renal stone
7. Renal failure

Investigations

1. Rectal exam
2. CBC with DC
3. Arterial blood gases
4. Uric acid
5. Prostate-specific antigen
6. ECG
7. Urinalysis and urinary culture with sensitivity testing
8. Ultrasonography of the kidney, ureter, and bladder
9. CT of pelvis

Red Flags

1. Indicate to the patient that you will perform a digital rectal examination now.
2. Tricyclic antidepressants can cause anuria. Therefore, a detailed drug history should be taken.
3. If you suspect renal failure, differentiate among prerenal, renal, and postrenal failure.

Case 32   ### Differential Diagnoses

1. Pneumonia
2. Pericarditis
3. Bronchitis
4. Pneumothorax
5. Congestive heart failure
6. Autoimmune disease
7. Tuberculosis

Investigations

1. CBC with DC
2. Vitamin B_{12}, thiamine levels
3. Blood glucose
4. Hemoglobin 1ac
5. Chest x-ray
6. Blood culture
7. Echocardiography

Red Flags

1. Counsel the patient about blood glucose control. Indicate the importance of taking medications, proper diet control, and regular exercise.
2. Counsel the patient about the adverse effects of alcohol. The history must include the CAGE questions.

Case 33   Differential Diagnoses

1. Community-acquired pneumonia
2. *Pneumocystis carinii* pneumonia (now *P. jiroveci*)
3. Tuberculosis
4. Histoplasmosis
5. Tumor
6. Coccidioidomycosis

Investigations

1. CD4 count
2. CBC with DC
3. Chest x-ray
4. CT of chest
5. Blood culture
6. Sputum culture
7. Purified protein derivative test for TB

Red Flags

1. Counsel the patient about the importance of safe sexual practices.
2. Indicate the importance of regular medical checkups and prophylactic medication use to prevent the further progression of disease.

Case 34   Differential Diagnoses

1. MI
2. Pulmonary embolism
3. Angina
4. Pneumothorax
5. Pneumonia
6. Aortic dissection
7. Gastroesophageal reflux disease
8. Trauma

Investigations

1. ECG
2. Cardiac enzymes
3. Chest x-ray
4. V/Q scan
5. Arterial blood gases
6. Echocardiography
7. CBC with DC

Red Flags

1. Elderly women with a history of recent surgery, deep vein thrombosis, oral contraceptive use, and immobility are at higher risk for pulmonary embolism.
2. Smoking, hyperlipidemia, diabetes mellitus, age, male sex, and type A personality are risk factors for myocardial infarction.

Case 35   **Differential Diagnoses**

1. Meningitis
2. Encephalitis
3. Brain abscess
4. Brain tumor
5. Tension headache
6. Endocarditis
7. Alcohol withdrawal

Investigations

1. Lumbar puncture
2. CT
3. ELISA/Western blot test
4. CBC with DC
5. Blood culture
6. Vitamin B_{12}, thiamine
7. Urine toxicology screen
8. Serum toxicology screen

Red Flags

1. Counsel the patient about the aspects of alcohol use.
2. If the patient gives a history of intravenous drug use, you must look for track marks. Common areas for track marks are the cubital fossa and around the ankle.
3. If you suspect IV drug use, consent for HIV testing must be obtained before performing an ELISA or Western blot test.

Bonus Case

You may be asked to fill out a form for a mini-mental status exam. You should use the Folstein Mini-Mental Status Exam (maximum score = 30).

Orientation to Time (1 pt each)

- What year is this?
- What season is this?
- What month is this?
- What is today's date?
- What day of the week is it?

Orientation to Place (1 pt each)

- Which state are we in?
- What county are we in?
- What city are we in?
- Which hospital are we in?
- Which floor are we on?

Immediate Recall (3 pts)

- Name three objects and ask the patient to repeat all three objects. Repeat the three objects until the patient learns them all. Record the number of times it take the patient to learn the objects.

Attention (either test) (5 pts)

- Serial 7s: Tell the patient, "Subtract 7 from 100, then subtract 7 from the answer you get, and keep subtracting 7 until I tell you to stop."
- Ask the patient to spell the word "world" backward.

Delayed Recall (3 pts)

- Ask the patient, "What are the three words I asked you to remember earlier?"

Naming (2 pts)

- Show the patient common objects (e.g., wristwatch and pen) and ask the patient to name them.

Repetition (1 pt)

- Have the patient repeat the following sentence exactly:
- "No ifs, ands, or buts."

3-Stage Command (3 pts)

- Have the patient listen first and then follow these directions when you are finished: "Take it in your right hand, use both hands to fold it in half, and then put it on the floor."

Reading (1 pt)

- Tell the patient to read and follow these commands:
- "Close your eyes."

Copying (1 pt)

- Give the patient a clean sheet of paper and ask him/her to copy a design.

Writing (1 pt)

- On the same sheet of paper, ask the patient to write a complete sentence.

MODEL CASE

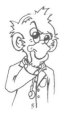

11

An example of a practice case is presented below. We have included everything right from the first knock on the door to the closing handshake. If you follow these steps, you will have no problem in conquering the USMLE Step 2-CS.

"SPs, please prepare," is what you hear on the intercom. At this point you should take a deep breath. You should be relaxed and remain confident because you know that you have prepared well. Unfortunately, it is premature to think about what you will do after the exam. That may take place around case 8 or 9.

About 2 minutes later you will hear, "You may begin your encounter." The next step is to make your cheat sheet. Don't hesitate to draw your lines. If you need to write down your mnemonics, this is the time to do it. Next you open the encounter box on the doorway. Let us say it reads as follows:

> Mrs. Jane Smith is 52 years old. She presents to your office with severe substernal chest pain that radiates to her left shoulder for the past 3 hours.
> Her vital signs are as follows:
> Pulse: 92 beats/minute
> BP: 146/94 mm Hg
> Respirations: 26/minute
> Temperature: 100.1°F
> Take a proper history, perform a physical examination, and write the patient note.

Before you enter the room to begin your encounter, there are a few things you should do:

> 1. Try to recall your differential diagnoses and the list of investigations. You may jot them down if you want.
> 2. You should come up with a game plan that includes which systems you are going to examine. In this case you are thinking cardiovascular and respiratory systems and perhaps the abdomen.
> 3. Last, but probably most important, take another deep breath.

This entire process should take no more than 45 to 60 seconds once the second bell has sounded.

Knock on the door, and enter with a smile.

Dr.: *"Good morning Mrs. Smith. I am Dr. ABC* (make sure that you shake hands with the SP). *It's nice to meet you. I am here to ask you a few questions and then perform a physical exam. If you're feeling cold, would you like me to drape you?"* (Wait for an answer. Go ahead and drape the patient if appropriate, then begin the HPI.)

"So what brings you in today?" (Remember to facilitate the interview.)

Pt.: "Well, I have had this pain in my chest for the past couple of hours, I have been sweating and short of breath. I am worried that I am going to die."

"Well, Mrs. Smith, it is too early for me to tell you if you are going to die. Let me complete my history and physical exam, run a couple of tests, and then we will go from there. Can you show me with a finger exactly where it hurts?"

"The pain is around the center of my chest, more so on the left side."

"On a scale of 10, 1 being the least and 10 being the worst, how would you grade the pain?"

"I'd say about an 8."

"What does the pain feel like?"

"What do you mean? It's pain and it hurts bad!"

"I mean, Mrs. Smith, would you say the pain is stabbing, burning, or crushing in nature?"

"Oh, I'd say it's a squeezing type pain."

"When did this start?"

"I told you earlier that it began a couple of hours ago!"

This is a very controversial question. The reason is that the SP stated already when the pain started, but our recommendations are still to ask the question. In this particular scenario, just apologize and continue.

"Does the pain move anywhere?"

"It goes to my left shoulder."

"Anywhere else?"

"No."

"Have you noticed anything that makes the pain better?"

"When I rest."

"Anything that makes it worse?"

"When I walk."

"Do you feel nauseated, or did you vomit? Did you have any fever, headache, or shortness of breath?" (Don't bombard the patient with multiple questions like this. Ask them one at a time.)

"Do you feel nauseated?"

"I do feel nauseous, and for some reason I have been sweating profusely."

"Any vomiting?"

"No."

"Any fever?"

"No."

"Headache?"

"No."

"Mrs. Smith, I am going ask you a few questions about your past medical health."

"Okay."

"Have you ever experienced this type of pain in the past?"

"No."

"Are you allergic to any food or medications?"

"I am allergic to penicillin."

"And what does it do?"

"Well, I get hives, rashes, and chills."

"Are you currently taking any medications?"

"I take a laxative for my constipation."

"Anything else?"

"Some ginseng and some gingko for my memory."

"Have you ever had a high blood pressure or diabetes?"

"Not that I know of."

"Have you had any surgery before?"

"I had my appendix removed about 20 years ago."

"Any problems in defecating or urinating?"

"I don't understand what you mean?"

"I'm sorry. I meant do you have any difficulties in passing bowel movements or going to the bathroom?"

"No."

You might get stumped in a situation like this, but remember not to use medical terminology with the SP. If a situation such as this arises during your encounter, just rephrase the question using common language and continue.

"How are you sleeping these days?"

"Just fine."

"Now, Mrs. Smith, I am going to ask you some personal questions. Let me assure you that whatever we discuss will remain confidential. Is that alright with you?"

"Yes, it is."

"Are you sexually active?"

"Yes, with my husband of 23 years."

"When was your last period?"

"About 3 years ago."

"When was your first period?"

"When I was 12 years old."

"How were your cycles?"

"They were very regular, and I had minimal cramps."

"Have you ever been pregnant?"

"Yes, two wonderful boys."

"What was the mode of delivery?"

"Normal vaginal."

"Any complications during childbirth, or any miscarriages?"

"No."

"Mrs. Smith, I am no going to ask you about your personal life. Do you use tobacco, either smoke or chewed?"

"Yes, I have been smoking cigarettes for the past 26 years."

"How many packs a day?"

"Almost two per day."

You can counsel the patient about the cessation of smoking either now or after the physical examination. Our recommendation is that it be done at the end, so you can combine the counseling and closing in one session.

"Do you drink alcohol?"

"Only on occasion."

"How often is an occasion?"

"I have a glass or two of wine on the weekend."

"Do you use any recreational or illicit drugs?"

"No."

"Have you every used any form of intravenous drugs?"

"Never."

"Are you currently employed?"

"I manage a day care center."

"Now I'd like to know a little about your family. Has anyone in your family ever had the same symptoms that you are having now?"

"Not that I can remember."

"Has anyone in your family ever been diagnosed or treated for any medical or surgical illness?"

"Yes, my father had hypertension. He died of a heart attack 5 years ago. My mother died of breast cancer 4 years ago."

You must remember to counsel the patient about breast cancer. Inform the patient about different screening modalities.

"Have you traveled anywhere recently?"

"I went to Cleveland and Chicago last month."

"Have you traveled anywhere internationally?"

"No."

"Is your vaccination schedule up to date?"

"Why yes, I just had my last tetanus booster 2 months ago."

"Mrs. Smith, excuse me while I wash my hands."

While you wash your hands, you should be thinking of which systems to examine. In this case both respiratory and cardiovascular systems should be examined. Also by this point your cheat sheet should be on the verge of completion.

"Now, Mrs. Smith, I need to take a look at your chest. May I untie your gown?"

"Yes, you may."

"I am now going to feel your chest. Tell me if you feel any pain."

"Okay, go ahead."

"I am now going to feel your heart."

"Okay."

"I am going to tap your chest."

"Okay."

"Can you lift your right arm so I can tap your right side?"

"Okay."

"Can you lift your left arm so I can tap your left side?"

"Okay."

"I am now going to tap your back."

"Okay."

"Mrs. Smith, I am going to listen to your heart."

"Okay."

"Can you please lift your left breast so I can listen to your heart."

"Yes, I can."

"Now I am going to listen to your lungs. I want you to take a deep breath in and out."

"Alright."

"Okay, Mrs. Smith. Can I help you tie up your gown?"

"Yes, you may."

At this point in time your cheat sheet should be complete. You should have approximately 2-3 minutes remaining in your encounter. Your closing consists of reading your cheat sheet to the SP.

"Well, Mrs. Smith, you told me that you had chest pain for the past couple of hours. Now I am thinking of a couple of different things. You may have suffered a heart attack or are suffering from heartburn, but to confirm that, I need to get an ECG done."

"What is an ECG?"

"We attach some stickers with wires running to a monitor that records your heart activity."

"Okay."

"I am also going to need a blood sample so I can get a complete blood work-up with the level of your heart enzymes and the level of your electrolytes."

"Wow, you can get all of that from a blood sample?"

Pain in chest for few hours
    Grade 8
    Squeezing
    Past few hours
    Radiates to left shoulder
    Associated with walking
    Relieved by rest
    Sweating, nausea
	Myocardial infarction
	    Unstable angina
	    Tension pneumothorax
	    Carditis
	    Pneumonia
	    Aortic dissection
	    Pulmonary embolism
	    _____
	    _____
	    Smoking
	    Breast cancer

First time
    Penicillin
    Laxatives
    Appendectomy * 20 years ago
    NL: urination and defecation, sleep
    Married
    2 children, vaginal delivery
    First menstrual period age 12, regular
    Menopause * 3 years ago
    Smokes 2-3 packs/day * 26 years
    Occasional drinker
    Father: hypertension
    Mother: died d/t breast cancer
    Up-to-date with vaccinations
	ECG
	    Cardiac enzymes (CPK-MB, troponin)
	    Chest x-ray
	    CBC with DC
	    Electrolytes
	    Echocardiography

"Yes, Mrs. Smith. It is also possible that you may have problems with your lungs. You may have air or fluid between your lungs and the membrane covering them. Therefore I need to get a chest x-ray. That would also rule out pneumonia."

"Now, Mrs. Smith, you did tell me that you have smoked 2–3 packs of cigarettes for the last 26 years. Do you know that you are killing your lungs and yourself?"

"Yes, I do. I've tried to quit, but I haven't been able to. You know how hard it is."

"Well, that is a common complaint among patients. But there are ways to quit. There are medications that reduce the craving as well as nicotine patches that can help. Also there are support groups that can help you quit."

"Really! I never knew."

"Would you be interested?"

"I would."

"Great. After we finish with your current situation, we will further discuss your treatment options. Mrs. Smith, you also told me that your mother passed away due to breast cancer."

"Yes, I did."

"Mrs. Smith, when was your last mammogram?"

"I can't remember."

"Well, Mrs. Smith, just as a routine investigation I would like to get a mammogram done for you."

"Do you think that I have cancer?"

"I can't tell at this time. But I can tell you that breast cancer does run in the family. So just to be on the safe side, I would like to get this done."

"Whatever you say."

Look over your cheat sheet to make sure that you have covered everything. If you left anything out, now is the time to ask the SP.

"If you have any further questions at this time I would be more than happy to answer them."

"Well, I think that's it, doc."

(While shaking hands): *"Thank you for your cooperation, Mrs. Smith. It was nice meeting you, and I'll be back when your results are in. Take care, and bye for now."*

12

APPENDIX

COMMON MEDICAL ABBREVIATIONS

- **yo** years old
- **m** male
- **f** female
- **b** black
- **w** white
- **L** left
- **R** right
- **hx** history
- **h/o** history of
- **c/o** complaining of
- **NL** normal limits
- **WNL** within normal limits
- **BP** blood pressure
- **HR** heart rate
- **R** respirations
- **T** temperature
- **Ø** without or no
- **+** positive
- **−** negative
- **Abd** abdomen
- **AIDS** acquired immunodeficiency syndrome
- **AP** anteroposterior
- **B/L** bilateral
- **BS** bowel sounds
- **BUN** blood urea nitrogen
- **CABG** coronary artery bypass grafting
- **CBC** complete blood cell count
- **CCU** cardiac care unit
- **CHF** congestive heart failure
- **cig** cigarettes
- **COPD** chronic obstructive pulmonary disease
- **CPR** cardiopulmonary resuscitation
- **CT** computed tomography
- **CVA** cerebrovascular accident
- **CVAT** costovertebral angle tenderness
- **CVP** central venous pressure
- **CXR** chest x-ray
- **DM** diabetes mellitus
- **DTR** deep tendon reflexes
- **ECG** electrocardiogram
- **ED** emergency department
- **EMT** emergency medical technician
- **ENT** ears, nose, and throat
- **EOM** extraocular muscles
- **ETOH** alcohol
- **Ext** extremities
- **FH** family history
- **FOBT** fecal occult blood test
- **FSBS** fingerstick blood sugar
- **GI** gastrointestinal
- **GU** genitourinary
- **HEENT** head, eyes, ears, nose, and throat
- **HIV** human immunodeficiency virus
- **HTN** hypertension
- **IM** intramuscularly
- **IV** intravenously
- **JVD** jugular venous distention
- **KUB** kidney, ureter, and bladder
- **LMP** last menstrual period
- **LN** lymph nodes
- **LP** lumbar puncture
- **MI** myocardial infarction
- **MRI** magnetic resonance imaging
- **MVA** motor vehicle accident
- **N.** normal
- **Neuro** neurologic
- **NIDDM** non-insulin-dependent diabetes mellitus
- **NKA** no known allergies
- **NKDA** no known drug allergy
- **NSR** normal sinus rhythm
- **NVBS** normal vesicular breath sounds
- **PA** posteroanterior
- **PERLA** pupils equal, react to light and accommodation
- **PMI** point of maximal impulse
- **po** orally
- **Pt.** patient
- **PT** prothrombin time
- **PTT** partial thromboplastin time
- **RBCs** red blood cells
- **ROM** range of motion
- **SH** social history
- **TIA** transient ischemic attack
- **TM** tympanic membrane
- **U/A** urinalysis
- **URI** upper respiratory tract infection
- **WBCs** white blood cells

CHEAT SHEET MODEL

History of Presenting Illness	Differential Diagnoses

Counseling & Red Alerts in Doorway Information

Past Medical History

Investigations

SAMPLE PATIENT NOTE PAGE

History

Include significant positives and negatives from history of present illness, past medical history, review of system(s), social history, and family history.

Physical Examination

Indicate only pertinent positive and negative findings related to the patient's chief complaint.

Differential Diagnoses

1.
2.
3.
4.
5.

Investigations

1.
2.
3.
4.
5.

Summary of Recommendations for Adult Immunization

Adapted from the recommendations of the Advisory Committee on Immunization Practices (ACIP)* by the Immunization Action Coalition, July 2004

Vaccine name and route	For whom it is recommended	Schedule for routine and "catch-up" administration	Precautions and contraindications (mild illness is not a contraindication)
Influenza Trivalent inactivated influenza vaccine (TIV) *Give IM* Live attenuated influenza vaccine (LAIV) *Give intranasally*	• All adults who are 50yrs of age or older. • People 6m–50yrs of age with medical problems (e.g., heart disease, lung disease, diabetes, renal dysfunction, hemoglobinopathies, immunosuppression) and/or people living in chronic-care facilities. • People (≥6m of age) working or living with at-risk people. • Women who will be pregnant during the influenza season. • All health care workers and other persons who provide direct care to at-risk people. • Household contacts and out-of-home caregivers of children ages 0–23m. • Travelers at risk for complications of influenza who go to areas where influenza activity exists or who may be among people from areas of the world where there is current influenza activity (e.g., on organized tours). • Persons who provide essential community services. • Students or other persons in institutional settings (e.g., those who reside in dormitories). • Anyone wishing to reduce the likelihood of becoming ill with influenza. **Special Notes on the use of influenza vaccines** • Inactivated influenza vaccine may be given to any person ≥6 months of age for whom the vaccine is not contraindicated. Live attenuated influenza vaccine may be given to healthy, non-pregnant persons 5–49 years of age for whom the vaccine is not contraindicated. • Use of inactivated influenza vaccine is preferred for persons in close contact with severely immunosuppressed persons during periods when the immunocompromised person requires a protective environment (e.g., persons with bone marrow transplants).	• Given every year. • October through November is the *optimal* time to receive annual influenza vaccination to maximize protection. • Influenza vaccine may be given at any time during the influenza season (typically December through March) or at other times when the risk of influenza exists. • May give with all other vaccines.	• Previous anaphylactic reaction to this vaccine, to any of its components, or to eggs. • Moderate or severe acute illness. • Do not give live attenuated influenza vaccine to persons ≥50 years of age, pregnant women, or to persons who have: asthma, reactive airway disease or other chronic disorder of the pulmonary or cardiovascular systems; an underlying medical condition, including metabolic diseases such as diabetes, renal dysfunction, and hemoglobinopathies; a known or suspected immune deficiency disease or who are receiving immunosuppressive therapy; a history of Guillain-Barré syndrome. • See Special Notes in columns 2–3 regarding who may not receive LAIV.
Pneumococcal polysaccharide (PPV23) *Give IM or SC*	• Adults who are 65yrs of age or older. • People 2–64yrs of age who have chronic illness or other risk factors, including chronic cardiac or pulmonary diseases, chronic liver disease, alcoholism, diabetes mellitus, CSF leaks, candidate for or recipient of cochlear implant, as well as people living in special environments or social settings (including Alaska Natives and certain American Indian populations). Those at highest risk of fatal pneumococcal infection are people with anatomic asplenia, functional asplenia, or sickle cell disease; immunocompromised persons including those with HIV infection, leukemia, lymphoma, Hodgkin's disease, multiple myeloma, generalized malignancy, chronic renal failure, or nephrotic syndrome; persons receiving immunosuppressive chemotherapy (including corticosteroids); and those who received an organ or bone marrow transplant. Pregnant women with high-risk conditions should be vaccinated if not done previously.	• Routinely given as a one-time dose; administer if previous vaccination history is unknown. • One-time revaccination is recommended 5yrs later for people at highest risk of fatal pneumococcal infection or rapid antibody loss (e.g., renal disease) and for people ≥65yrs of age if the 1st dose was given prior to age 65 and ≥5yrs have elapsed since previous dose. • May give with all other vaccines.	• Previous anaphylactic reaction to this vaccine or to any of its components. • Moderate or severe acute illness. **Note:** Pregnancy and breastfeeding are not contraindications to the use of this vaccine.
Hepatitis B (Hep B) *Give IM* Brands may be used interchangeably.	• All adolescents. • High-risk adults, including household contacts and sex partners of HBsAg-positive persons; users of illicit injectable drugs; heterosexuals with more than one sex partner in 6 months; men who have sex with men; people with recently diagnosed STDs; patients receiving hemodialysis and patients with renal disease that may result in dialysis; recipients of certain blood products; health care workers and public safety workers who are exposed to blood; clients and staff of institutions for the developmentally disabled; inmates of long-term correctional facilities; and certain international travelers. **Note:** Prior serologic testing may be recommended depending on the specific level of risk and/or likelihood of previous exposure. **Note:** In 1997, the NIH Consensus Development Conference, a panel of national experts, recommended that hepatitis B vaccination be given to all anti-HCV positive persons. **Ed. note:** Provide serologic screening for immigrants from endemic areas. When HBsAg-positive persons are identified, offer appropriate disease management. In addition, screen their sex partners and household members and, if found susceptible, vaccinate.	• Three doses are needed on a 0, 1, 6m schedule. • Alternative timing options for vaccination include 0, 2, 4m and 0, 1, 4m. • There must be 4wks between doses #1 and #2, and 8wks between doses #2 and #3. Overall there must be at least 16wks between doses #1 and #3. • **Schedule for those who have fallen behind:** If the series is delayed between doses, DO NOT start the series over. Continue from where you left off. • May give with all other vaccines.	• Previous anaphylactic reaction to this vaccine or to any of its components. • Moderate or severe acute illness. **Note:** Pregnancy and breastfeeding are not contraindications to the use of this vaccine.
Hepatitis A (Hep A) *Give IM* Brands may be used interchangeably.	• People who travel outside of the U.S. (except for Western Europe, New Zealand, Australia, Canada, and Japan). • People with chronic liver disease, including people with hepatitis C; people with hepatitis B who have chronic liver disease; illicit drug users; men who have sex with men; people with clotting-factor disorders; people who work with hepatitis A virus in experimental lab settings (not routine medical laboratories); and food handlers when health authorities or private employers determine vaccination to be cost effective. **Note:** Prevaccination testing is likely to be cost effective for persons >40yrs of age as well as for younger persons in certain groups with a high prevalence of hepatitis A virus infection.	For Twinrix™ (hepatitis A and B combination vaccine [GSK]) three doses are needed on a 0, 1, 6m schedule. • Two doses are needed. • The minimum interval between dose #1 and #2 is 6m. • If dose #2 is delayed, do not repeat dose #1. Just give dose #2. • May give with all other vaccines.	• Previous anaphylactic reaction to this vaccine or to any of its components. • Moderate or severe acute illness. • Safety during pregnancy has not been determined, so benefits must be weighed against potential risk. **Note:** Breastfeeding is not a contraindication to the use of this vaccine.

Summary of Recommendations for Adult Immunization (continued)

Vaccine name and route	For whom it is recommended	Schedule for routine and "catch-up" administration	Precautions and contraindications (mild illness is not a contraindication)
Td (Tetanus, diphtheria) *Give IM*	• All adolescents and adults. • After the primary series has been completed, a booster dose is recommended every 10yrs. Make sure your patients have received a primary series of 3 doses. • A booster dose as early as 5yrs later may be needed for the purpose of wound management, so consult ACIP recommendations.* • Use Td, not tetanus toxoid (TT), for all indications.	• Give booster dose every 10yrs after the primary series has been completed. • For those who are unvaccinated or behind, complete the primary series (spaced at 0, 1–2m, 6–12m intervals). Don't restart the series, no matter how long since the previous dose. • May give with all other vaccines.	• Previous anaphylactic or neurologic reaction to this vaccine or to any of its components. • Moderate or severe acute illness. **Note:** Pregnancy and breastfeeding are not contraindications to the use of this vaccine.
MMR (Measles, mumps, rubella) *Give SC*	• Adults born in 1957 or later who are ≥18yrs of age (including those born outside the U.S.) should receive at least one dose of MMR if there is no serologic proof of immunity or documentation of a dose given on or after the first birthday. • Adults in high-risk groups, such as health care workers, students entering colleges and other post–high school educational institutions, and international travelers, should receive a total of two doses. • Adults born before 1957 are usually considered immune but proof of immunity may be desirable for health care workers. • All women of childbearing age (i.e., adolescent girls and premenopausal adult women) who do not have acceptable evidence of rubella immunity or vaccination. • Special attention should be given to immunizing women born outside the United States in 1957 or later.	• One or two doses are needed. • If dose #2 is recommended, give it no sooner than 4wks after dose #1. • May give with all other vaccines. • If varicella vaccine and MMR are both needed and are not administered on the same day, space them at least 4wks apart. • If a pregnant woman is found to be rubella-susceptible, administer MMR postpartum.	• Previous anaphylactic reaction to this vaccine or to any of its components. • Pregnancy or possibility of pregnancy within 4 weeks (use contraception). • Persons immunocompromised because of cancer, leukemia, lymphoma, immunosuppressive drug therapy, including high-dose steroids or radiation therapy. **Note:** HIV positivity is NOT a contraindication to MMR except for those who are severely immunocompromised. • If blood, plasma, and/or immune globulin were given in past 11m, see ACIP statement *General Recommendations on Immunization** regarding time to wait before vaccinating. • Moderate or severe acute illness. **Note:** Breastfeeding is not a contraindication to the use of this vaccine. **Note:** MMR is not contraindicated if a tuberculin skin test (i.e., PPD) was recently applied. If PPD and MMR not given on same day, delay PPD for 4–6wks after MMR.
Varicella (Var) (Chickenpox) *Give SC*	All susceptible adults and adolescents should be vaccinated. It is especially important to ensure vaccination of the following groups: susceptible persons who have close contact with persons at high risk for serious complications (e.g., health care workers and family contacts of immunocompromised persons) and susceptible persons who are at high risk of exposure (e.g., teachers of young children, day care employees, residents and staff in institutional settings such as colleges and correctional institutions, military personnel, adolescents and adults living with children, non-pregnant women of childbearing age, and international travelers who do not have evidence of immunity). **Note:** People with reliable histories of chickenpox (such as self or parental report of disease) can be assumed to be immune. For adults who have no reliable history, serologic testing may be cost effective since most adults with a negative or uncertain history of varicella are immune.	• Two doses are needed. • Dose #2 is given 4–8wks after dose #1. • May give with all other vaccines. • If varicella vaccine and MMR are both needed and are not administered on the same day, space them at least 4wks apart. • If the second dose is delayed, do not repeat dose #1. Just give dose #2.	• Previous anaphylactic reaction to this vaccine or to any of its components. • Pregnancy or possibility of pregnancy within 4 weeks (use contraception). • Persons immunocompromised because of malignancies and primary or acquired cellular immunodeficiency including HIV/AIDS. (See *MMWR* 1999, Vol. 48, No. RR-6.) **Note:** For those on high-dose immunosuppressive therapy, consult ACIP recommendations regarding delay time.* • If blood, plasma, and/or immune globulin (IG or VZIG) were given in past 11m, see ACIP statement *General Recommendations on Immunization** regarding time to wait before vaccinating. • Moderate or severe acute illness. **Note:** Breastfeeding is not a contraindication to the use of this vaccine. **Note:** Manufacturer recommends that salicylates be avoided for 6wks after receiving varicella vaccine because of a theoretical risk of Reye's syndrome.
Polio (IPV) *Give IM or SC*	Not routinely recommended for persons 18yrs of age and older. **Note:** Adults living in the U.S. who never received or completed a primary series of polio vaccine need not be vaccinated unless they intend to travel to areas where exposure to wild-type virus is likely. Previously vaccinated adults can receive one booster dose if traveling to polio endemic areas.	• Refer to ACIP recommendations* regarding unique situations, schedules, and dosing information. • May give with all other vaccines.	• Previous anaphylactic or neurologic reaction to this vaccine or to any of its components. • Moderate or severe acute illness. **Note:** Pregnancy and breastfeeding are not contraindications to the use of this vaccine.
Meningococcal *Give SC*	Vaccinate people with risk factors. Discuss disease risk and vaccine availability with college students. Consult ACIP statement* on meningococcal disease (6/30/00) for details.		

* For specific ACIP immunization recommendations, refer to the statements, which are published in *MMWR*. To obtain a complete set of ACIP statements, call (800) 232-2522, or to access individual statements, visit CDC's website: www.cdc.gov/nip/publications/ACIP-list.htm or visit IAC's website: www.immunize.org/acip This table is revised yearly because of the changing nature of U.S. immunization recommendations. Visit the Immunization Action Coalition's website at www.immunize.org/adultrules to make sure you have the most current version. We extend our thanks to William Atkinson, MD, MPH, from CDC's National Immunization Program, and Linda Moyer, RN, from the Division of Viral Hepatitis, at CDC's National Center for Infectious Diseases for their assistance. This table is published by the Immunization Action Coalition, 1573 Selby Avenue, St. Paul, MN 55104, (651) 647-9009. Email: admin@immunize.org

www.immunize.org/catg.d/p2011b.pdf • Item #P2011 (7/04)

Recommended Childhood and Adolescent Immunization Schedule
United States · July–December 2004

| | Range of Recommended Ages | | | | | Catch-up Immunization | | | | Preadolescent Assessment | | |

Vaccine ▼ / Age ▶	Birth	1 mo	2 mo	4 mo	6 mo	12 mo	15 mo	18 mo	24 mo	4-6 y	11-12 y	13-18 y
Hepatitis B[1]	HepB #1	only if mother HBsAg(-)									HepB series	
			HepB #2			HepB #3						
Diphtheria, Tetanus, Pertussis[2]			DTaP	DTaP	DTaP		DTaP			DTaP	Td	Td
Haemophilus influenzae Type b[3]			Hib	Hib	Hib	Hib						
Inactivated Poliovirus			IPV	IPV		IPV				IPV		
Measles, Mumps, Rubella[4]						MMR #1				MMR #2	MMR #2	
Varicella[5]						Varicella					Varicella	
Pneumococcal[6]			PCV	PCV	PCV	PCV				PCV	PPV	
Influenza[7]						Influenza (Yearly)				Influenza (Yearly)		
Vaccines below red line are for selected populations												
Hepatitis A[8]										Hepatitis A Series		

This schedule indicates the recommended ages for routine administration of currently licensed childhood vaccines, as of April 1, 2004, for children through age 18 years. Any dose not given at the recommended age should be given at any subsequent visit when indicated and feasible. ▨Indicates age groups that warrant special effort to administer those vaccines not previously given. Additional vaccines may be licensed and recommended during the year. Licensed combination vaccines may be used whenever any components of the combination are indicated and the vaccine's other components are not contraindicated. Providers should consult the manufacturers' package inserts for detailed recommendations. Clinically significant adverse events that follow immunization should be reported to the Vaccine Adverse Event Reporting System (VAERS). Guidance about how to obtain and complete a VAERS form can be found on the Internet: www.vaers.org or by calling 800-822-7967.

1. Hepatitis B (HepB) vaccine . All infants should receive the first dose of hepatitis B vaccine soon after birth and before hospital discharge; the first dose may also be given by age 2 months if the infant's mother is hepatitis B surface antigen (HBsAg) negative. Only monovalent HepB can be used for the birth dose. Monovalent or combination vaccine containing HepB may be used to complete the series. Four doses of vaccine may be administered when a birth dose is given. The second dose should be given at least 4 weeks after the first dose, except for combination vaccines which cannot be administered before age 6 weeks. The third dose should be given at least 16 weeks after the first dose and at least 8 weeks after the second dose. The last dose in the vaccination series (third or fourth dose) should not be administered before age 24 weeks.

Infants born to HBsAg-positive mothers should receive HepB and 0.5 mL of Hepatitis B Immune Globulin (HBIG) within 12 hours of birth at separate sites. The second dose is recommended at age 1–2 months. The last dose in the immunization series should not be administered before age 24 weeks. These infants should be tested for HBsAg and antibody to HBsAg (anti-HBs) at age 9–15 months.

Infants born to mothers whose HBsAg status is unknown should receive the first dose of the HepB series within 12 hours of birth. Maternal blood should be drawn as soon as possible to determine the mother's HBsAg status; if the HBsAg test is positive, the infant should receive HBIG as soon as possible (no later than age 1 week). The second dose is recommended at age 1–2 months. The last dose in the immunization series should not be administered before age 24 weeks.

2. Diphtheria and tetanus toxoids and acellular pertuss is (DTaP) vaccine . The fourth dose of DTaP may be administered as early as age 12 months, provided 6 months have elapsed since the third dose and the child is unlikely to return at age 15–18 months. The final dose in the series should be given at age ≥4 years. *Tetanus and di phthe ria toxoi ds (Td)* is recommended at age 11–12 years if at least 5 years have elapsed since the last dose of tetanus and diphtheria toxoid-containing vaccine. Subsequent routine Td boosters are recommended every 10 years.

3. Haemoph ilus inf luenzae type b (Hib) conjugate vaccine. Three Hib conjugate vaccines are licensed for infant use. If PRP-OMP (PedvaxHIB or ComVax [Merck]) is administered at ages 2 and 4 months, a dose at age 6 months is not required. DTaP/Hib combination products should not be used for primary immunization in infants at ages 2, 4 or 6 months but can be used as boosters following any Hib vaccine. The final dose in the series should be given at age ≥12 months.

4. Measles, mumps, and rubella vaccine (MMR). The second dose of MMR is recommended routinely at age 4–6 years but may be administered during any visit, provided at least 4 weeks have elapsed since the first dose and both doses are administered beginning at or after age 12 months. Those who have not previously received the second dose should complete the schedule by the visit at age 11–12 years.

5. Varicella vaccine. Varicella vaccine is recommended at any visit at or after age 12 months for susceptible children (i.e., those who lack a reliable history of chickenpox). Susceptible persons age ≥13 years should receive 2 doses, given at least 4 weeks apart.

6. Pneumococcal vaccine. The heptavalent **pneumococcal conjugate vaccine (PCV)** is recommended for all children age 2–23 months. It is also recommended for certain children age 24–59 months. The final dose in the series should be given at age >12 months. **Pneumococcal polysaccharide vaccine (PP**V**)** is recommended in addition to PCV for certain high-risk groups. See *MMWR* 2000;49(RR-9):1-35.

7. Influenza vaccine. Influenza vaccine is recommended annually for children aged ≥6 months with certain risk factors (including but not limited to asthma, cardiac disease, sickle cell disease, HIV, and diabetes), healthcare workers, and other persons (including household members) in close contact with persons in groups at high risk (see *MMWR* 2004;53;[RR-6]:1-40) and can be administered to all others wishing to obtain immunity. In addition, healthy children aged 6–23 months and close contacts of healthy children aged 0–23 months are recommended to receive influenza vaccine, because children in this age group are at substantially increased risk for influenza-related hospitalizations. For healthy persons aged 5–49 years, the intranasally administered live, attenuated influenza vaccine (LAIV) is an acceptable alternative to the intramuscular trivalent inactivated influenza vaccine (TIV). See *MMWR* 2004;53;[RR-6]:1-40. Children receiving TIV should be administered a dosage appropriate for their age (0.25 mL if 6–35 months or 0.5 mL if ≥3 years). Children aged ≤8 years who are receiving influenza vaccine for the first time should receive 2 doses (separated by at least 4 weeks for TIV and at least 6 weeks for LAIV).

8. Hepatitis A vacci ne. Hepatitis A vaccine is recommended for children and adolescents in selected states and regions and for certain high-risk groups; consult your local public health authority. Children and adolescents in these states, regions, and high-risk groups who have not been immunized against hepatitis A can begin the hepatitis A immunization series during any visit. The 2 doses in the series should be administered at least 6 months apart. See *MMWR* 1999;48(RR-12):1-37.

For additional information about vaccines, including precautions and contraindications for immunization and vaccine shortages, please visit the National Immunization Program Web site at www.cdc.gov/nip/ or call the National Immunization Information Hotline at 800-232-2522 (English) or 800-232-0233 (Spanish).

Approved by the Advisory Committee on Immunization Practices (www.cdc.gov/nip/acip), the American Academy of Pediatrics (www.aap.org), and the American Academy of Family Physicians (www.aafp.org).

Birth to 36 months: Boys
Length-for-age and Weight-for-age percentiles

NAME _____

RECORD # _____

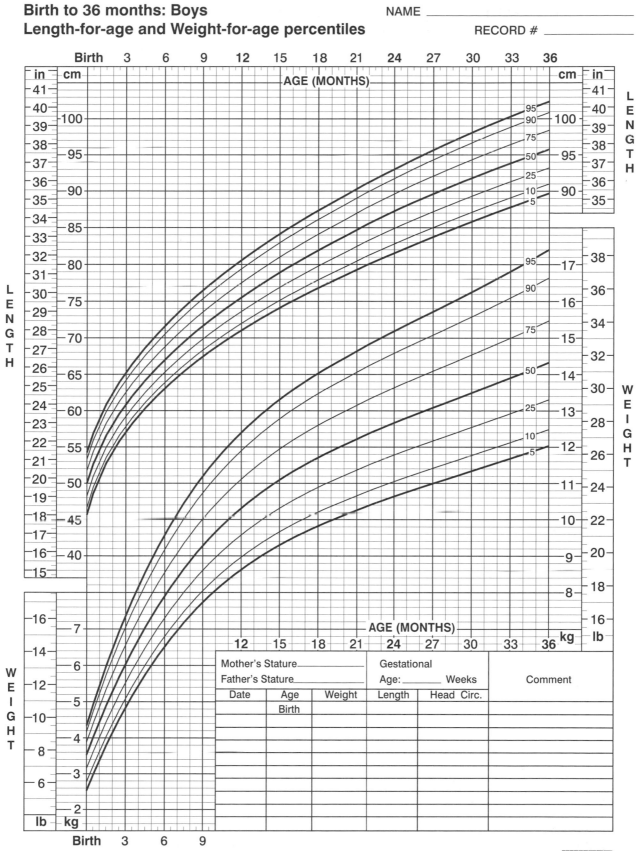

Published May 30, 2000 (modified 4/20/01).

SOURCE: Developed by the National Center for Health Statistics in collaboration with
the National Center for Chronic Disease Prevention and Health Promotion (2000).
http://www.cdc.gov/growthcharts

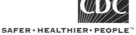

SAFER · HEALTHIER · PEOPLE™

2 to 20 years: Boys
Stature-for-age and Weight-for-age percentiles

NAME

RECORD #

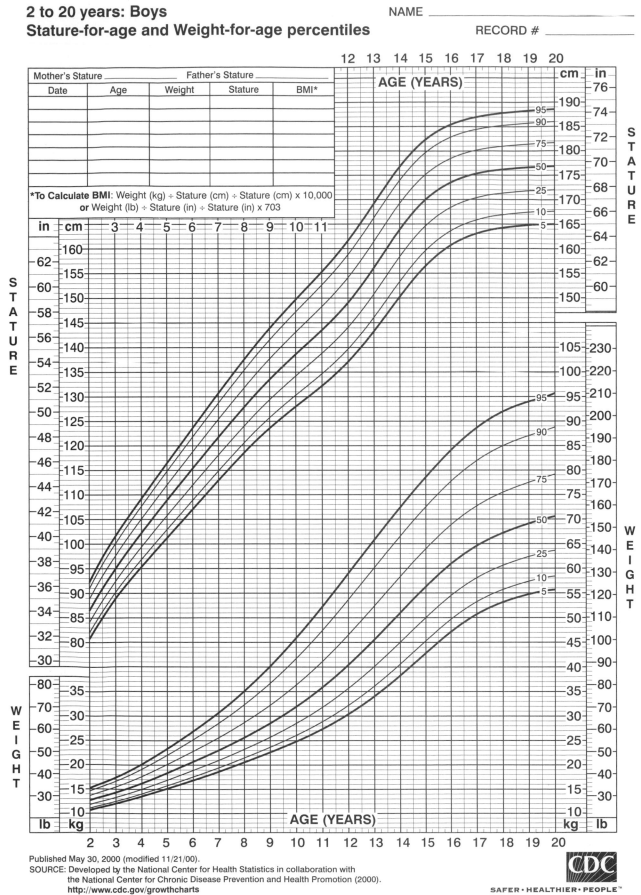

Mother's Stature _____ Father's Stature _____

Date	Age	Weight	Stature	BMI*

*To Calculate BMI: Weight (kg) ÷ Stature (cm) ÷ Stature (cm) x 10,000
or Weight (lb) ÷ Stature (in) ÷ Stature (in) x 703

Published May 30, 2000 (modified 11/21/00).
SOURCE: Developed by the National Center for Health Statistics in collaboration with
the National Center for Chronic Disease Prevention and Health Promotion (2000).
http://www.cdc.gov/growthcharts

CDC

SAFER · HEALTHIER · PEOPLE™

INDEX

A

Abbreviations, 151–152
ABCDEFGHIJK, 10
Abdominal exam, 24–25, 39
Abdominal fullness, 117, 136–137
Abdominal pain, 62, 79–82, 114, 132
Abducent nerve, 26
Abortion, 94
Acne, 104–105, 121
Activities of daily living, 12
AIDS, 73–74, 119, 139
AIDS, 119, 139
Alcohol use, 14, 120, 140
Altered mental status, 67–68, 110,
    127–128
Amenorrhea, 88, 99
Anion gap increase, 106, 123
Anterior drawer sign, 29
Appetite loss, 81–82
Asterexis, 29
Auscultation
    abdominal, 24
    heart, 22
    lungs, 23–24

B

Babinski reflex, 27
Back pain, 45–47
Bad breath, 83–84
Bad news, 34
Bipolar disorder, 101
Bleeding
    nasal, 52–53, 65
    postcoital, 89
    rectal, 53–54
Blood, urinary, 105, 121–122
Blurred vision, 55–56
Breast
    enlargement of, 116, 135
    lump in, 108, 125
Breath, shortness of, 105, 110, 114, 122, 128,
    133
Breathing difficulty, 96–97
Brudzinski's sign, 29

C

CAGE, 14
Cardiovascular exam, 21–22, 39
Carpal tunnel syndrome, 68–69
CASE THIS IF MORPHINE JOKE,
    11
Central nervous system exam, 25–28, 39
Cerebellar assessment, 28
Cervical discharge, 62
Chadwick's sign, 99

Cheat sheet, 37–38, 152
Checklist, 19–21
Chest
    examination of, 23–24
    pain in, 3, 43–45
Cigarette smoking, 15, 111, 129
Compassion, 40
Consciousness
    clouding of, 115, 134
    loss of, 115, 133–134
Constipation, 61
Convulsions, 71
Costovertebral angle, 25
Cough, 50–52
Counseling, 31–32
Cranial nerve exam, 26
Crash diet, 98
Cyclothymic disorder, 101

D

Deep tendon reflexes, 27
Depression, patient history of, 11
Diarrhea, 63, 66–67, 111, 129–130
Dieting, 98
Domestic abuse, 82–83
DR. ABCDEFGHI, 10–11
Dyspareunia, 74–75

E

Ear
    discharge from, 116, 134–135
    exam of, 28–29, 39
Edema, leg, 118, 137
Eyes
    exam of, 28, 39
    red, 112, 130
    yellowness of, 60

F

Facial droop, 113, 131
Facial nerve, 26
Facial pain, 87
Falls, 69–70
Family history, 15
Fatigue, 65, 70, 77
Female exam, 63–64
Fever, 64–65, 71, 79–80
Finger-to-nose test, 28

G

Genital ulcers, 112, 131
Glossopharyngeal nerve, 26
Growth charts, 157–158

H

Hand pain, 68–69, 117, 136
Head exam, 28, 39
Headache, 64–65, 66, 109, 127
Hearing loss, 106, 123–124
Hearing voices, 100
Heart exam, 22
Heel-to-knee test, 28
HEENT exam, 28–29, 39
Hegar's sign, 99
Hematemesis, 94–95
Heroin use, 111, 129
Hiccups, 84–85
HIV infection, 73–74, 119, 139
Hoarseness, 85–86
Homan's sign, 29
Hypertension, 78–79, 114–115, 119, 120,
    133–134, 138, 139
Hypoglossal nerve, 26

I

Immunization
    adult, 154–155
    childhood, 156
Impotence, 86
Insomnia, 77–78
Inspection
    abdominal, 24
    cardiovascular, 22
    chest, 23
Instability, 92
Interview, 12–17
    about bad news, 34
    closing of, 35
    excessive talking and, 32
    introduction of, 12–13
    patient history in, 13–17
    patient questions during, 32–33
    telephone, 33
Itching, 95–96

J

Jaundice, adult, 60
    pediatric, 75–76

K

Kernig's sign, 29
Knee pain, 47–48, 49–50

L

Leg
    pain in, 109, 126–127
    swelling of, 118, 137
    ulcers of, 62

LIQOR DRAW, 9
Liver, palpation of, 25
Loss of consciousness, 115, 133–134
Lunch break, 7
Lung exam, 22–24
Lymphadenopathy, 108, 126

M

Malar pain, 66
Memory loss, 67–68, 120, 140–141
Menstruation, 88
Mental deterioration, 67–68
Mental status, altered, 67–68, 110, 127–128
Mental status exam, 25–26
Mini-Mental Status Exam, 140–141
Mitral valve prolapse, 113, 132
Model case, 143–149
Mood disorders, 101
    patient history of, 11
Moses sign, 29
Motor exam, 26–27
Motor vehicle accident, 96–97
Murphy's sign, 29
Musculoskeletal exam, 40

N

Nasal discharge, 66
Nausea, 60, 64–65
Nose
    bleeding from, 52–53, 65
    exam of, 29, 39

O

Obturator sign, 29
Oculomotor nerve, 26
Olfactory nerve, 26
Optic nerve, 26
Orientation, 5–6

P

PACK BUSH SOS (MODELS) FTV,
    9–10
Pain
    abdominal, 62, 79–80, 80–82, 114, 132
    back, 45–47
    chest, 3, 43–45
    facial, 87
    hand, 68–69, 117, 136
    knee, 47–50
    leg, 109, 126–127
    malar, 66
    shoulder, 48–49
Palpation
    abdominal, 25
    cardiovascular, 22
    chest, 23
Palpitations, 56–57
Past medical history, 9–10, 13–15
Pathological reflex, 27
Patient history, 9–17
    activities of daily living in, 12
    of depression, 11

Patient history (*Continued*)
    of past medical history, 9–10, 13–15
    of presenting illness, 9, 13
    of trauma, 10–11
    pediatric, 10, 15–16
    psychiatric, 11, 16–17
Patient note, 37–40, 153
Pediatric patient history, 10, 15–16
Percussion
    abdominal, 24
    cardiovascular, 22
    chest, 23
Personal history, 14
Phalen's test, 29
Photophobia, 64–65
Physical exam, 19–30
    abdominal, 24–25, 39
    cardiovascular, 21–22, 39
    central nervous system, 25–28, 39
    checklist for, 19–21
    HEENT, 28–29, 39
    musculoskeletal, 29–30, 40
    respiratory, 22–24, 39
PICCLE, 38
Postcoital bleeding, 89
Posterior drawer sign, 29
Pre-employment screening (NASA), 108,
    125
Pregnancy, 99
Presenting illness, 9, 13
Psoas sign, 29
Psychiatric exam, 40
Psychiatric patient history, 11, 16–17
Psychosis, 100

R

Rash, 71
Rebound tenderness, 25
Rectal bleeding, 53–54
Recurrent abortion, 94
Red eyes, 112, 130
Reflexes, 27
Registration, 5
Respiratory exam, 22–24, 39
Rinne's test, 29

S

SAVED, 11
Scoring, 2–3
Sensory exam, 27–28
Sexual assault, 93
Sexual history, 14
SHEATH DRAFT, 12
Short stature, 76
Shortness of breath, 105, 110, 114, 122, 128,
    133
Shoulder pain, 48–49
Sickle cells, 107, 124–125
SIGE CAPS, 11
Singultus, 84–85
Sinusitis, 64–65
Sleeping difficulty, 70, 77–78
Smoking, history, 15
Smoking, counseling, 111, 129

Snoring, 107, 124
Spinal accessory nerve, 26
Spleen, palpation of, 25
Standardized patient, 2
    challenges of, 32–34
Step 2 Clinical Skills (Step 2–CS) exam, 1–3
    cheat sheet for, 37–38, 152
    fifteen-minute periods of, 6–7
    history taking in, 9–17
    orientation for, 5–6
    patient note in, 37–40
    physical environment for, 6
    physical exam in, 19–30
    registration for, 5
    thought process for, 3
Straight leg raising test, 29
Substance use, 14, 111, 129
Suicide, 97–98
Superficial reflex, 27
Swallowing difficulty, 89–90

T

Tachypnea, 65
Tactile fremitus, 23
Telephone interview, 33
Throat exam, 29, 39
Tinel's sign, 29
Tobacco use history, 15
Transillumination test, 29
Trauma, patient history of, 10–11
Tremors, 57–59
Trigeminal nerve, 26
Trochlear nerve, 26

U

Ulcers
    genital, 112, 131
    leg, 62
Unsteadiness, 92
Urinary frequency, 91
Urine
    absence of, 118, 137–138
    blood in, 105, 121–122

V

Vaccination
    adult, 154–155
    childhood, 156
Vagal nerve, 26
Vaginal discharge, 59
Vestibulocochlear nerve, 26
Vision
    blurred, 55–56
    loss of, 109, 127
Voice strain, 85–86
Vomiting, 54–55, 60, 79–80

W

Weber's test, 29
Websites, 2
Weight gain, 72–73
Weight loss, 71–72, 89–90, 111, 129–130